HIGHLAND Dancing

The textbook
of the
Scottish Official Board
of Highland Dancing

LINDSAY
PUBLICATIONS

Highland Dancing
the Textbook of the Scottish Official Board of Highland Dancing.
© **Scottish Official Board of Highland Dancing**
Sixth Edition (1993)

Reprinted 1996, 2001, 2004, 2006

Published by
Lindsay Publications
PO Box 812
Glasgow G14 9NP

ISBN 1 8981 6901 2

Text design by Stuart Nichols
Illustrations by Maggie Scott, with amendments by David Wilson
Cover design by Smith & Paul Associates, Glasgow

Printed and Bound by Bell and Bain Ltd., Glasgow

CONTENTS

Foreword   v

Introduction   vi

Chapter One: Basic Positions and
**   Basic Movements**   1
General Remarks and Preliminary
    Definitions   1

A: Basic Positions
1. *Foot Positions*   1
Definitions   1
Preliminary Remarks   1
The line of Direction   2
First Position   3
Second Position   3
Second Aerial Position   4
Third Position   5
Third Aerial Position   5
Third Rear Position   6
Third Rear Aerial Position   6
Third Crossed Position   7
Fourth Position   7
Fourth Aerial Position   8
Fourth Rear Position   8
Mid-Fourth Position   8
Mid-Fourth Aerial Position   8
Fourth Intermediate Position   9
Fourth Intermediate Aerial Position   9
Fourth Intermediate Rear Position   10
Fourth Intermediate Rear Aerial
    Position   10
Fourth-opposite-Fifth Position   11
Fourth-opposite-Fifth Rear Position   11
Fifth Position   12
Fifth Rear Position   12

2. *Arm Positions*   13
Grouping of Fingers   13
First Position   13
Second Position   14
Third Position   14
Fourth Position   15
Fifth Position   15

3. *Head Positions*   16
First Position   16
Second Position   16

B: Basic Movements   17
The Bow   17
Hop   18
Spring   18
Step   18
Assemble   18
Disassemble   18
Change   19
Leap   20
Brush   21
Shake   21
Pas de Basque   22
Open Pas de Basque   22
High Cut   23
High Cut in Front   24
Balance   24
Travelling Balance   24
Rock   25
Round-the-Leg   26
Shedding   26
Toe-and-Heel   26
Heel-and-Toe   26
Back-Stepping   26
Shuffle   27
Spring Point   27
Pivot Turn   28
Hop-Brush-Beat-Beat   28
Shake-Shake-Down   28
Propelled Pivot Turn or Reel Turn   29
Progressive Strathspey Movement   29
Progressive Reel Movement   30

C: Basic Steps   30

Chapter Two: Highland Dances   31
1: The Highland Fling   31
2: The Sword Dance (Gillie Chalium)   34
3: Seann Triubhas   40
4: Strathspey   48
5: Highland Reel   50
6: Basic Reel Steps   51
7: Reel of Tulloch or "Hullachan"   54

Chapter Three: Rudiments of Music   57
Counting of Highland Dancing Steps
    or Movements to Music   58

FOREWORD

The Forewords to previous editions of this textbook were written by Brigadiers Harry Clark and Alasdair Maclean, sadly no longer with us. With their great love of Highland Dancing they would, I am sure, be delighted and impressed to see how the Scottish Official Board has grown in stature and command over the years. This textbook is in many ways a tribute to the foresight of those two fine Highland gentlemen and to the many teachers, judges, dancers and administrators who saw the need for a democratically elected governing body for Highland Dancing and who then went on to provide the framework within which a definitive textbook of our traditional Scottish art could be produced.

To transfer the poetry of music and movement into pages of text is a most difficult task. To try to describe in precise mathematical terms and plain English the smooth free-flowing movement of dance steps is almost impossible. Since the first edition of *Highland Dancing* was printed there have been many amendments to the text. The majority of changes have been required to meet unexpected interpretations of the given descriptions, not to alter the movements described. Over the years refinements of language have helped to reduce this problem but a textbook still cannot replace a good instructor whose aim must be to guide students through the mechanics of movement to the feeling behind it, and this textbook should therefore be used as a guide and reference volume by both teacher and student.

The textbook *Highland Dancing* has been an incredible success, not just in Scotland but all over the world. It has enabled young people in many different countries to enjoy our colourful heritage in the knowledge that they were using the same steps and technique as the dancers 'Back Home' in Scotland. The advantages gained have become more obvious as communications and modern methods of travel have allowed dancers to fly regularly to and fro between provinces, states and countries, taking part in demonstrations and competitions. No longer is it possible to label a competitor as Australian, South African, Canadian or American because of the steps used or differences in technical approach. Indeed, it seems the Scots must look to their laurels as top flight dancers from all of those countries are now competing and winning at the major championships in Scotland.

At last we have a truly international appreciation of the definitive finer points of Highland Dancing, an international community of Scottish Dancers working for and with one another towards even higher standards of excellence.

I trust this volume will give you pleasure, that it will produce solutions for any questions you may have and that it will become a friend to you in your search for that supreme level of excellence to which we all aspire.

Billy Forsyth, Chairman S.O.B.H.D.

INTRODUCTION

In any particular country the evolution of a national form of dancing is bound to give rise to diverse opinions as to the correct method of performing that country's traditional dances unless it is controlled by some one generally recognised authority. Many of the innovations which have periodically appeared in Highland Dancing were accepted by dancers all over Scotland, but certain brilliant exponents of the art have, from time to time, introduced new ideas and variations of their own. These new ideas were adopted only by the pupils and followers of those who invented them, and there has developed a chaotic situation, in which our traditional dances are danced differently in different parts of our country. Dancers competing at the various games throughout Scotland have had to vary their style and alter their steps according to the district in which they were competing, or according to the known stylistic preferences of the judges before whom they were appearing.

Various associations of teachers, and many individuals well versed in Highland Dancing, have compiled their own descriptions of our traditional dances, and their own versions of the traditional technique. Some of these accounts of Highland Dancing resemble one another fairly closely, but no two of them are exactly alike.

To the organisers of Highland Games, that part of the programme which was concerned with Highland Dancing was a constant thorn in the flesh. Complaints were continually being made to them about bad or biased judging, or about unsatisfactory features in the conduct of the competitions; and there is no doubt that an appreciable percentage of those complaints was justified. Yet the organisers could do little or nothing about them, because there was no generally recognised authority to which they could refer such complaints for consideration and necessary action. Nor was there any body to which competitors having a legitimate grievance against the organisers of, or the judges at, any particular Games could appeal, because the rules laid down by the promoters of any particular competition were not applicable to other competitions, and there were no generally applicable rules governing the conduct of championships or other competitions of lesser importance.

Towards the end of the year 1949 the Scottish Dance Teachers' Alliance made a move towards bringing this unsatisfactory state of affairs to an end, by advocating the establishment of a representative board of control. The principal aims and objects of the board would be to stabilise the technique of Highland Dancing, to formulate laws and regulations covering every aspect of the art, and to do everything in its power to further the interests of our national dancing. It was fitting that this first move should have been made by the Alliance, because it is the only association of professional teachers of dancing which can, by reason of its constitution, claim to be purely Scottish. Getting in touch with other associations which foster Highland Dancing, and with various organisations which sponsor Highland Games, the Alliance invited each of these bodies to send delegates to a meeting specially convened for the purpose of considering the advisability of establishing a representative body to control Highland Dancing. Many prominent personalities, well known to the public as exponents (past or present), as judges, or as patrons, of Highland Dancing, but not connected with any professional association, were also invited to attend this meeting. Mr James Adam having kindly offered, for this purpose, the Plaza Ballroom in Stirling, the meeting took place there in January 1950. It was presided over by Mr Jack Muir, who was President of the Alliance at that time, and resulted in the inauguration of 'The Scottish Official Board of Highland Dancing'.

This Board is representative of all organisations and individuals interested in any aspect of Highland Dancing, and its constitution makes provision for: four Office-Bearers, three delegates and one non-voting deputy each from Examining

Bodies, one Delegate and one non-voting Deputy each from Represented Members and Affiliated Members (Overseas Associations); one Delegate each from a limited number of Games Organisations; not more than ten Independent Members; and one non-voting delegate each from Associate Members.

This book sets forth the stabilised technique of Highland Dancing which has been compiled by the Board and adopted by all associations and individuals connected with that body. This is tantamount to stating that practically every qualified teacher of Highland Dancing in Scotland has adopted that technique.[1]

In every part of the world where Scots are to be found, and particularly in every part of the British Commonwealth, there is usually a Scottish Society of some description, and most of these societies are sponsors of Highland Dancing. As ambassadors for this branch of our national culture they look, naturally, to their mother country for guidance. Hitherto they have been in a quandary as to whose description of the Highland dances, and whose version of the technique, they should adopt. Now, with the advent of the Scottish Official Board of Highland Dancing, they have available to them authoritative, practical and comprehensive instructions governing that art in all its aspects.

---

[1] Originally it was intended also to provide a brief but authoritative account of the history of Highland Dancing. Gradually, however, it became clear that the difficulties in the way of such an attempt are at present well-nigh insuperable: reliable evidence concerning origins and early development is scarce and scattered; in the general neglect of Scottish culture which has prevailed, until recently, in all four Scottish universities, Highland Dancing has been largely ignored by learned men; and as yet little or no serious research has been done. There is an opportunity here for academic investigations which, it is to be hoped, they will not fail much longer to exploit.

Dedicated to Jack Muir
Chairman of the Scottish Official Board of Highland Dancing
until his death in December 1967,
whose technical skill and devotion to Highland Dancing
made this book possible

CHAPTER ONE: BASIC POSITIONS AND BASIC MOVEMENTS

General remarks and preliminary definitions

1 The body should be held in a natural easy manner without stiffness, strain or exaggeration.

2 The foot supporting the weight of the body is called the *Supporting Foot*. The other foot is called the *Working Foot*. While dancing, it is always the ball of the supporting foot that is in contact with the ground.

3 It should be the aim of the dancer to keep the supporting leg turned out at an angle of 45° to the line of direction (see p. 3), and the working leg turned out at an angle of not less than 45°, and in many cases 90° to the line of direction. This turning out of the knees tends to keep the apron of the kilt flat.

4 When executing any movement of elevation, the dancer should land on the count except where otherwise stated.

5 When the working foot has to be placed in or raised to any specified position whilst executing a movement of elevation, that foot arrives at the specified position simultaneously with the dancer landing on the supporting foot, unless otherwise stated.

6 *(a) Basic positions are the essential positions of the feet, arms and head on which all movements are founded.*

(b) A Basic Movement is the combining, by movement, of two or more basic positions.

(c) A Basic Step is a combination of basic movements.

A: Basic positions

1: *Foot positions*

In this book foot positions are described and illustrated as nearly as possible as they should appear in actual dancing.

Definitions

A *Closed position* is one in which the feet are either in contact with each other, or the working foot is touching the supporting leg. (An exception is third crossed position.)

An *Open position* is one in which the working foot is not in contact with the supporting foot or the supporting leg.

A *Ground position* is one in which both feet are in contact with the ground.

An *Aerial position* is one in which the working foot is off the ground.

A *Rear position* is one in which the working foot is to the rear of the supporting foot.

Preliminary remarks

There are five *basic ground positions* of the feet, namely, first position, second position, third position, fourth position and fifth position. In addition to these there are four *derived positions:* one, being a variation of third position is called 'third crossed position'; the other three variations of fourth position, are called 'fourth intermediate position', 'fourth-opposite-fifth position', and 'mid-fourth position'.

In a *ground position* the following terms are used in describing various methods of placing the working foot.

(a) Toe. When in contact with the ground, without pressure, in an open position with the instep arched, or in a closed position with the foot vertical, it is said to be *pointed* or placed on the *toe*. When the working foot is pointed in an open position the knee of the working leg is kept straight except when placed in fourth-opposite-fifth position (see page 11).

(b) Half point. When the pads of the first two or three toes are in contact with the ground, with the ball of the foot off the ground, it is said to be placed on the *half point*.

1

When placed on the half point in an open position, the instep of the working foot should be arched with the knee of the working leg slightly relaxed; in a closed position, the working foot should be kept as vertical as possible.

When the working foot is placed on the half point, the weight of the body may be momentarily taken on it; the main weight being then retained on the other foot, thus providing the impetus for any required slight elevation or travel of that (i.e. the supporting) foot during the half point.

(c) *Ball.* When the pads of the toes and the ball of the foot are in contact with the ground with the instep arched, it is said to be placed on the *ball,* and the knee of the working leg is kept as straight as possible, but *without strain,* to allow for freedom of movement.

When the working foot is placed on the ball, the weight of the body is transferred on to it, so that when the dancer travels while so placing the foot, a step is taken.

(d) *Heel.* When the heel is in contact with the ground, with the sole of the foot kept straight and inclined upwards, the working foot is said to be placed on the *heel.* The heel is always placed without pressure, except in the eighth Seann Triubhas step, in which the weight is momentarily taken on it.

When the working foot is placed on the heel in any open position except fourth-opposite-fifth, the knee of the working leg is kept straight.

Certain positions have *rear* and/or *aerial* equivalents. There is no rear or aerial equivalent to first position or to third crossed position. There is an aerial equivalent, but no rear equivalent to second position. Conversely there is a rear equivalent but no aerial equivalent to fourth-opposite-fifth position and to the fifth position. There is an aerial but no rear equivalent to mid-fourth position.

In a *rear position,* the working foot is never placed on the half point or the heel.

In an *open aerial position,* the knee of the working leg should be kept straight, and the working foot, with the instep well arched, is off the ground with the toe at the correct height in relation to the supporting leg, to give *normal* level (in line with the centre of the calf), high level (in line with the centre of the knee-cap), or *low* level (in line with the ankle.)

In the two *closed aerial positions,* namely third aerial position and third rear aerial position, the working foot is off the ground in contact with, and at the correct height in relation to the supporting leg to give *normal* level (foot vertical—heel in line with the hollow below the knee) or, in the case of third aerial position only, *low* level (foot vertical—toe at ankle height) or *very low* level.

Note: In all aerial positions (open or closed), normal level is to be understood where no particular height is specified.

When preparing for and/or landing from a step of elevation with the weight equally distributed on the balls of both feet in third or fifth position, the insteps should be as fully arched as possible, the heels equidistant from the ground, and the knees slightly relaxed.

The line of direction

The line of direction is an imaginary line on the ground, passing from front to back between the heels of the dancer when standing in first position. The angles of basic foot positions are measured from this line.

To ensure a correct line of travel when executing steps which travel sideways towards second position (e.g. the second and eighth Seann Triubhas steps), the working foot should be placed slightly forward or backwards, as the case may be, from second position to commence the travel.

First position

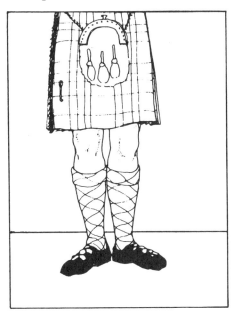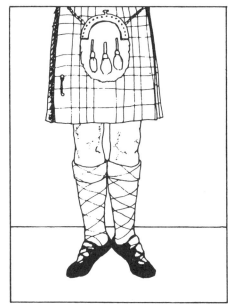

1/2

The heels are together, with the weight of the body equally distributed on both feet, which are turned out to form an angle of 90° (each foot being at an angle of 45° from the line of direction). The dancer may be standing with both feet flat on the ground (1), or may be poised on the balls of the feet (2).

Second position

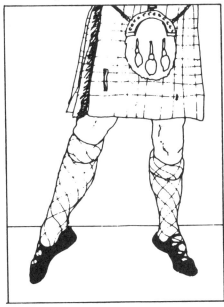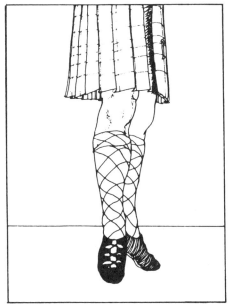

3/4

The working leg is extended directly to the side at an angle of 90° from the line of direction, the toe and heel of the working foot being in line with the heel of the supporting foot (4). The working foot may be placed on the toe (3), half point, ball, or heel and, except in the latter case, is placed approximately one and a half foot-lengths from the heel of the supporting foot.

Second aerial position

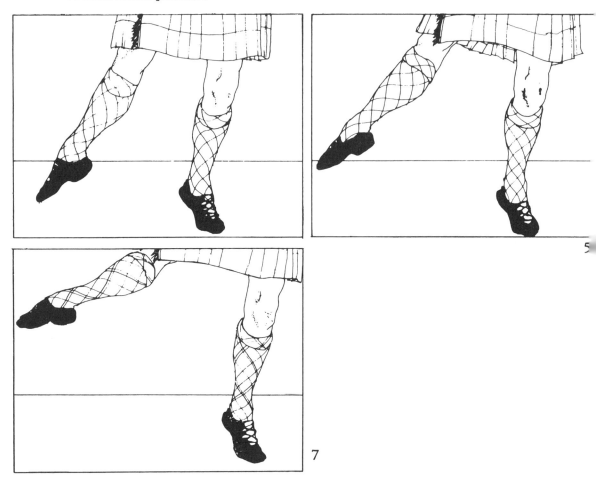

The working leg is extended to the side as in second position, but raised at the required level: low (5), normal (6), or high (7).

Third position

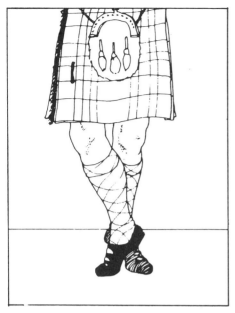 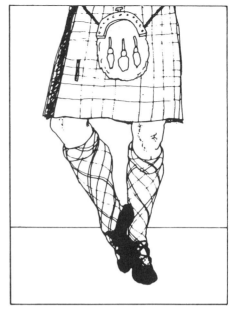

8/9

The working foot, which may be placed on the toe (9), half point, ball (8), or heel, touches the hollow of the supporting foot. When placed on the toe, half point, or heel, the working foot is turned out at an angle of 90° from the line of direction.

Note: When the weight of the body is equally distributed on the balls of both feet, the sole of the front foot is directly over the instep of the rear foot, both feet equally turned out at an angle of not less than 45° from the line of direction.

Third aerial position

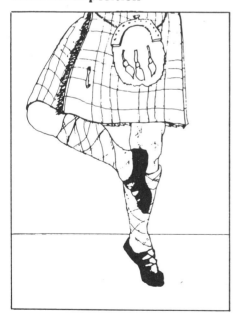

10

With the knee of the working leg pressed well back, the outside edge of the working foot is placed in contact with the front of the supporting leg, to give *normal* level with the heel slightly below the level of the knee cap of the supporting leg (10), *low* level with the toe in line with the ankle of the supporting leg or *very low* level with the foot slightly off the ground above third position.

5

Third rear position

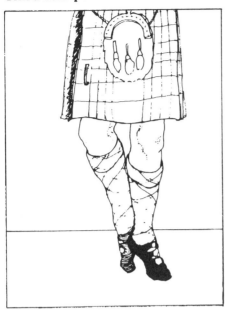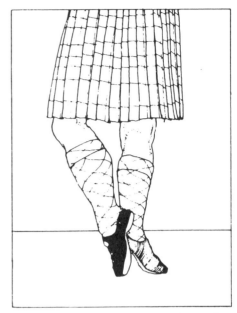

11/12

When placed on the toe, the hollow of the working foot touches the heel of the supporting foot. The working foot turned outwards at an angle of 90° from the line of direction.

Note: When placed on the ball the weight is equally distributed on the balls of both feet. The sole of the front foot is directly over the instep of the rear foot, both feet equally turned out at an angle of not less than 45° from the line of direction.

Third rear aerial position

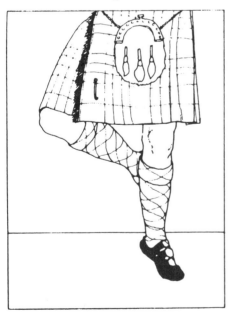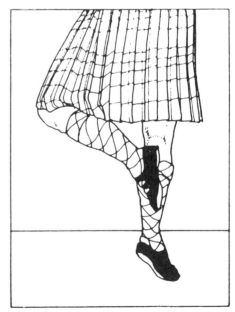

13/14

The working foot is placed behind the supporting leg at the same height as in third aerial position normal level, the inside edge of the foot being in contact with the calf of the supporting leg (14). The knee of the working leg is held well back, no part of the working foot being visible from the front (13).

6

Third crossed position

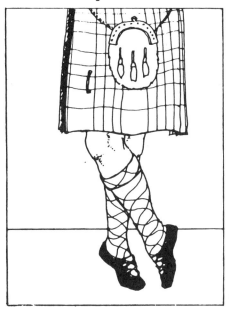

15

The working leg is crossed in front of the supporting leg with the half point of the working foot placed near the outside edge of the instep of the supporting foot or ball when used in the Highland Fling (15).

Fourth position

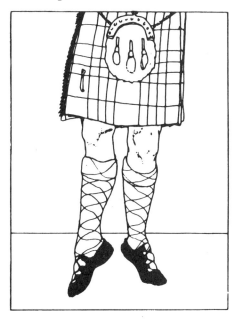

16

The working leg is extended to the front with both heels in line with the line of direction. The working foot, which is placed only on the toe or half point when used in the Sword Dance, is turned out at an angle of 45° from the line of direction (16).

Fourth aerial position

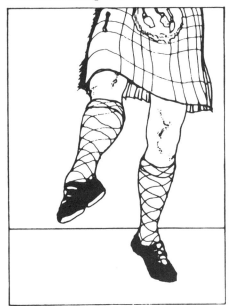

17

The working leg is extended to the front as in fourth position, but raised at the required level (17).

Fourth rear position
As in fourth position but the working foot is taken to the rear, and is placed on the ball or flat.

Mid-fourth position
The working leg is extended to the front, midway between fourth position and fourth intermediate position and is placed on the toe.

Mid-fourth aerial position
Extended to the front as for mid-fourth position and raised to low aerial.

Fourth intermediate position

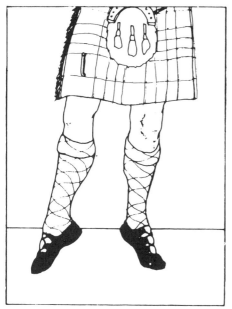

18

The working leg is extended diagonally forward at an angle of 45° from the line of direction with the working foot placed on the toe (18), half point or ball.

Fourth intermediate aerial position

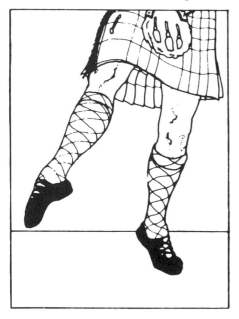

19

The working leg is extended as in fourth intermediate position, but raised at the required level (19).

Fourth intermediate rear position

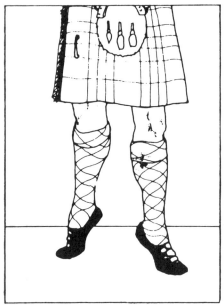

20

As in fourth intermediate position, but the working leg is extended to the rear and is placed only on the ball (20).

Fourth intermediate rear aerial position

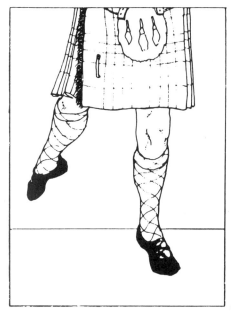

21

As in fourth intermediate rear position, but with the working leg raised at the required level (21).

Fourth-opposite-fifth position

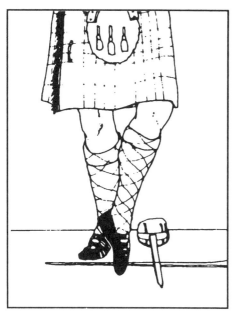

22

The working leg is extended to the front, but with the toe of the working foot in line with the heel of the supporting foot and with a slight relaxation of the knee of the working leg. The working foot may be placed on the toe (22), half point or heel and, in the latter case, the heel is placed in line with the toe joint of the supporting foot.
Note: This position is used only in the Sword Dance.

Fourth-opposite-fifth rear position
This is the position of the rear foot when the front foot is placed in fourth-opposite-fifth position.

Fifth position

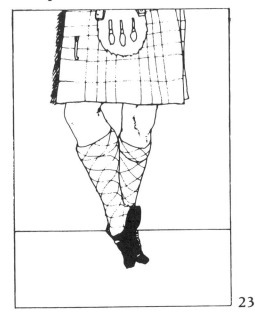

23

The working foot is in contact with the big toe joint of the supporting foot, and may be placed on the toe (23), half point, ball, or heel.

When placed on the toe, half point, or heel, the working foot faces outwards at an angle of 90° from the line of direction.

Note: When the weight of the body is equally distributed on the balls of both feet, the sole of the front foot is directly over the toes of the rear foot, both feet equally turned out at an angle of not less than 45° from the line of direction.

Fifth rear position

This is the position of the rear foot when it is placed on the ball and the front foot is in fifth position.

Grouping of fingers

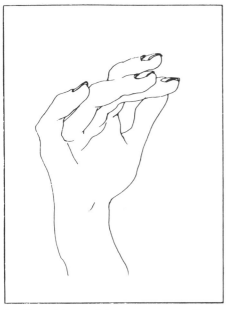

24

In all positions of the arms except first position, the fingers are lightly grouped and the thumb is in contact with the first joint of the middle finger (24).

First position
Both hands rest on the hips with the backs of the hands to the front, the knuckles facing the body with the wrists straight, and the elbows pointing directly out to the side (25).

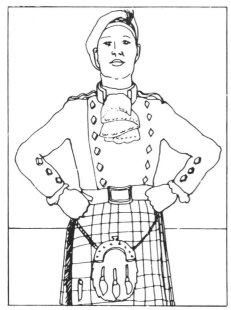

25

Note: When an arm is raised or lowered, there should be a minimum displacement of the elbow and no part of the arm or hand should come in front of the dancer's face. Exceptions are in the fourth bar of the introduction to the Seann Triubhas, where the hands come up in front of the face as the arms are raised in front of the body from fifth position, and also in the first and second Seann Triubhas steps when the arms are circled from first or fifth position.

Second position

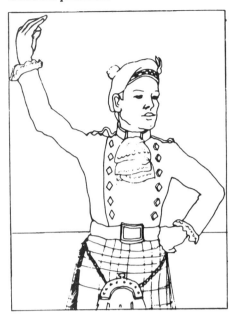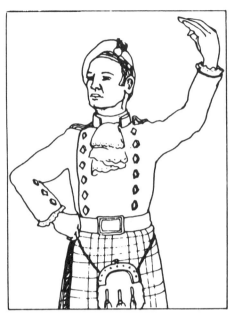

26/27

One arm is placed as in first position, the other is raised at the side, with the arm and wrist slightly curved, the hand slightly above and forward from the head-line, the palm turned inwards (26, 27).

Note: In this position the raised arm is always on the side opposite to the working leg, except in a propelled pivot turn.

Third position

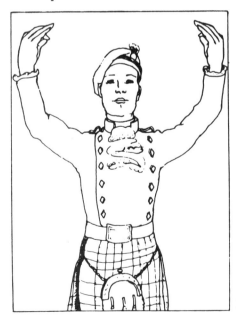

28

Both arms are placed as described for the raised arm in second position the palms facing inwards towards each other (28).

Fourth position

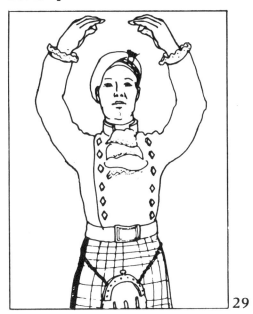

29

A closer and higher form of third position with the hands almost touching (29).

Fifth position
The arms are gently curved down in front of the body with the hands quite close to each other and the little fingers almost touching the kilt.

3: *Head Positions*

All head positions are described in relation to the position of the body.

First position

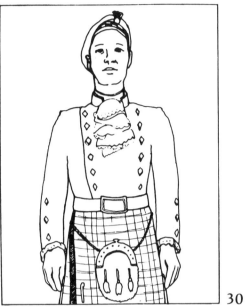

30

The head faces the front with the eyes level (30).

Note: The head is in first position when the arms are in first, third, fourth or fifth position, except when otherwise stated (30).

Second position

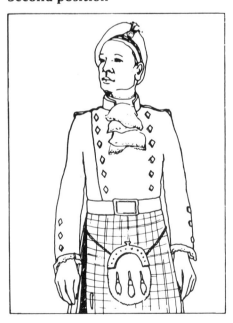 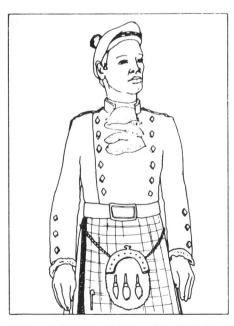

31/32

The head is directed diagonally to the right (31) or left (32), with the chin slightly raised.

Note: When the arms are in second position the head is turned away from the raised arm.

B: Basic movements

The system on which the counting of movements is based is explained in chapter three.

The bow

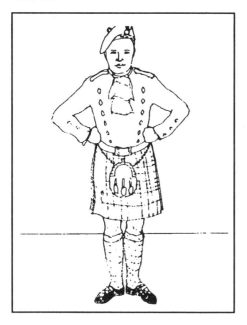

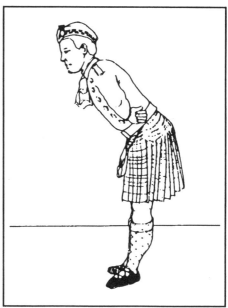

33/34

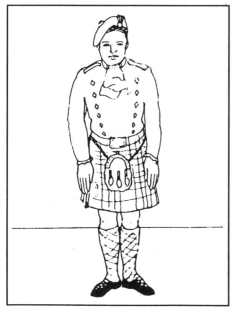

35

Stand with the feet and head in first position, arms by the side or in first position. Bow by inclining the body forward slowly, and return to the original position (33, 34, 35). If arms are by the sides, they should be taken to 1st position on the 1st count following the Bow, unless otherwise stated.

Note: The depth of the bow must not be exaggerated, and the count varies according to each dance, as described in chapter two.

Hop
A movement of elevation begun on the ball of one foot and finished by landing on the ball of the same foot.

Spring
As for hop, but landing on the ball of the other foot.

Step
A transfer of weight from one foot on to the ball of the other foot. Can be executed with or without travel and, where specially designated, the heel may be lowered to finish on the flat foot.

Assemble
A movement of elevation begun on the ball of one foot and finished by landing simultaneously on the balls of both feet in third or fifth position.

Disassemble
A movement of elevation begun in a closed position with the weight of the body equally distributed on the balls of both feet, and finished by landing on the ball of one foot with the other placed in, or raised to, a specified position.
Note: There is no travel on this movement, and, unless otherwise stated, during the elevation there is no extension of the foot upon which the dancer is to land.

Change

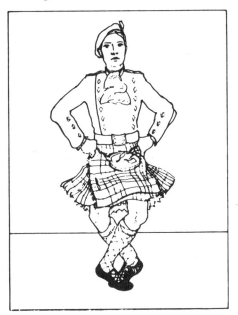

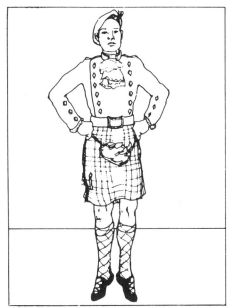

36/37

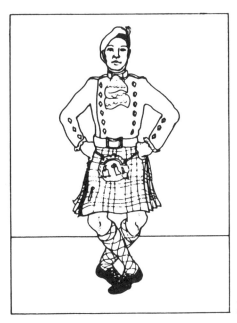

38

A movement of elevation begun with the weight of the body on the balls of both feet in fifth position and finished by landing on the balls of both feet simultaneously in fifth position with the other foot in front (36, 37, 38).

Note: During the elevation there is no extension towards second aerial position. This movement may also be executed using third position.

Leap

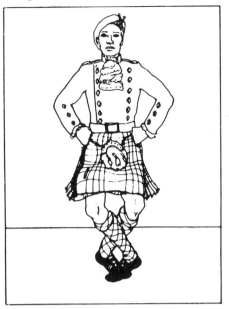 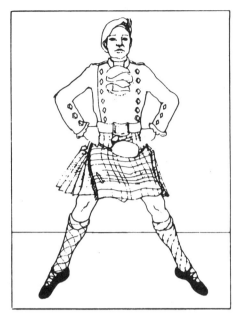

39/40

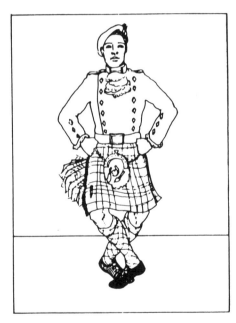

41

A movement of elevation begun from the balls of both feet in fifth position, extending both legs towards second aerial position, and finished by landing simultaneously on the balls of both feet in fifth position with or without change of feet (39, 40, 41).

Note 1: On the extension during the elevation, both legs should be straightened.

Note 2: This movement may also be executed using third position.

Brush

(a) *Outwards:* The half point of the working foot lightly touches the ground in its progress from third aerial position very low to an open aerial position or from a rear position, through first position to fourth aerial position.

(b) *Inwards:* The half point of the working foot lightly touches the ground in its progress from an open aerial position to an accepted closed position (see shuffle) or to third aerial position low (see hop-brush-beat-beat).

Note: When an outward brush is executed in conjunction with a spring or a hop, the working foot touches the ground almost simultaneously on landing.

Shake

A shake is always executed in conjunction with a hop.

(a) For *Seann Triubhas:* The working foot is progressively extended by two or more subsidiary movements (called shake actions) from third or fifth position to second aerial position high. The shake actions come from the knee controlled by the thigh and they should be started while flexing the knee of the supporting leg in preparation for the hop, simultaneously on landing from which, the working foot arrives at its highest point.

Example for counting: "and and a 1"

(b) For *Highland Fling:* The movement is always preceded by a placing of the working foot in third or fifth position from where it is extended to fourth intermediate aerial position using only one subsidiary movement. Thus, the actual shake movement consists of two shake actions, the first finished with the working foot in fourth intermediate aerial position low and the second with that foot arriving at fourth intermediate aerial position simultaneously on landing from the accompanying hop.

Examples for counting: (Including the preceding placing of the working foot.)

'1 and [and] a 2' or '1 [and] and a 2'.

Pas de Basque

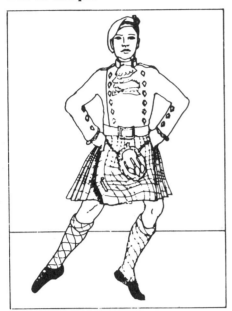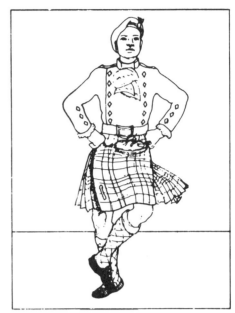

42/43

Preparing with an extension of the working foot to second aerial position low; spring to that side (42), bringing the new working foot to third or fifth position, placing it on the half point (43), then beat (without exaggeration) the ball of the other foot in third or fifth rear position, at the same time sharply extending the front foot, if required, to begin the next movement.

Note 1: The same position, third or fifth, must be used throughout the movement.

Note 2: When a turn, or part of a turn, is executed using two Pas de Basque, there is no extension to finish the first Pas de Basque, and the second is danced with little or no travel.

Note 3: This movement may also be danced with other than lateral travel, in which case the extension of the starting foot is along the required line of travel, generally towards fourth intermediate position.

Counting: (2 Pas de Basque)
Reel   1 & 2   3 & 4 = (2 bars)
Sword Dance   1& 2   3& 4 = (1 bar)

Open Pas de Basque

As in Pas de Basque, except that the front foot is placed in fourth-opposite-fifth position, and there is no extension at the finish.

Note: This movement is used only in the Sword Dance, and in the quick steps is also executed using fourth position, fourth intermediate position and second position.

High cut

Spring, hop or disassemble and, simultaneously on landing, take the working foot to third rear aerial position (44), then (working from the knee joint only) extend the working foot towards second aerial position (45) and return it to third rear aerial position (46). During the elevation one or both legs are extended towards second aerial position. Unless where specially designated, there is no side travel in this movement.

Note 1: Performed in series, high cutting can be described as a succession of springs from third rear aerial position to third rear aerial position , executing a high cut each time and during each elevation extending both feet towards second aerial position, although this extension of the foot from which each spring is commenced may be slight.

Note 2: If performed in a series, high cuts can be danced with or without extensions.

Note 3: In the Sword Dance and Reel where a series of extended high cuts are danced, the high cut which is executed in conjunction with the disassemble must be extended.

Note 4: Where a series of High Cuts are executed without extensions, it is permissible to extend a High Cut which is executed in conjunction with a disassemble.

High cut

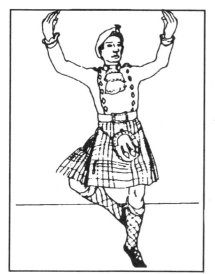 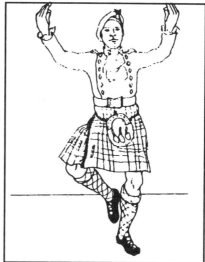

44/45

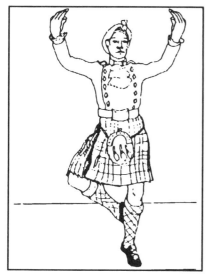

46

Counting: (four high cuts)

(a) To Strathspey tempo 1& 2& 3& 4&

In certain stated instances a single high cut may be counted 1 and [and]

(b) To Reel tempo 1 & 2 & 3 & 4 &

In certain stated instances, a single high cut may be counted 1 and [and]

High cut in front

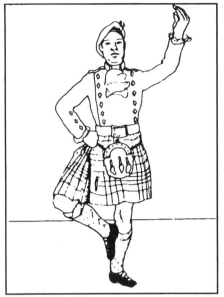

47

As for high cut, but the raised foot is taken through 4th intermediate aerial position to third aerial position (47) and the re-extension is towards fourth intermediate aerial position.
Note: High cuts in front are not performed in series, and in certain specified cases (e.g. in the sixth or ninth Seann Triubhas steps) the extensions are towards second aerial position.

Balance
Starting with one foot in the fourth intermediate aerial position and with the shoulder on the same side as the foot slightly advanced, spring on to that foot displacing the supporting foot which is taken to fourth intermediate rear aerial position. Repeat *contra* to complete the movement and finish in the starting position. This movement occupies two beats of music.

Travelling balance
Commence with the right foot in fourth intermediate aerial position, the body facing the front with the right shoulder slightly advanced, the *arms* in third position and the *head* in second position turned towards the front (48).
Bring the right foot inwards to take three steps RF, LF, RF, travelling diagonally backwards in a line approximately 45° to the line of direction , the foot positions being fifth position (49), fourth intermediate rear position (50) and fifth position (51), respectively, extending the left foot to fourth intermediate rear aerial position (simultaneously on taking the third step) (count '1 & 2'). The above is now repeated *contra*, travelling forward along the same diagonal line to finish the movement in the original starting position (48) (Count '3 & 4'). This movement can also be executed on the other side with the opposite foot and is invariably danced to the count '5 & 6, 7 & 8'.
Note: Throughout the movement, the upper part of the body is held erect.
Arms: The *arms* are taken inwards to fourth position during the backward travel then returned to third position during the forward travel or, alternatively, during the backward travel they are circled outwards and downwards at the sides to fifth position then, during the forward travel, they are circled outwards and upwards at the sides to third position.

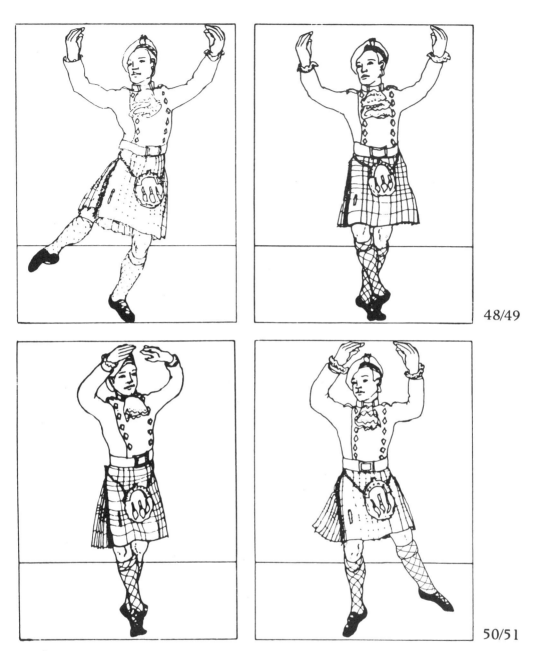

48/49

50/51

Rock

Spring from the third or fifth position to third rear position, or vice versa, pointing the working foot on landing. Rocks are usually danced in series, in which case the first rock may be executed starting from an open position. The rear foot is always pointed first.

Note: When the working foot is pointed during this movement the toe touches the ground lightly.

Round-the-leg

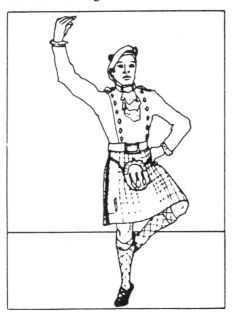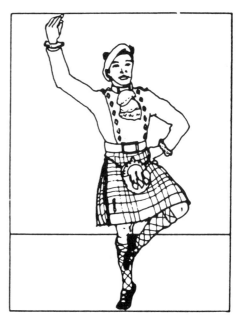

52/53

The working foot is passed from third rear aerial position (52) to third aerial position (53) or vice versa. During the movement the working foot must be kept as close as possible to the supporting leg with the knee of the working leg held well back.

Shedding

Hop, spring or disassemble pointing the working foot in second position (count '1'); hop, taking the working foot to third rear aerial position (count '2'); hop, executing a round-the-leg movement with the working foot to third aerial position (count '3'); hop, executing a round-the-leg movement with the working foot to third rear aerial position (count '4').

Note: Second position of the *arms* is invariably used with this movement, the raised arm being on the side opposite to the working foot.

Toe-and-heel

Hop or spring and, almost simultaneously on landing, point the working foot in a specified position, then hop and, almost simultaneously on landing, place the heel of the working foot in the same specified position. This movement occupies two beats of music.

Note 1: The toe and the heel must touch the ground lightly and the working foot must be kept fairly low.

Note 2: The specified position for this movement may be second, third, fourth-opposite-fifth or fifth. The 90° turn out required for the working foot in second position should also be aimed for in the other three positions.

Heel-and-toe

Hop, placing the heel of the working foot in second position; hop, pointing the working foot in third or fifth position. This movement occupies two beats of music.

Back-stepping

Starting with one foot in third aerial position, execute a round-the-leg movement to third rear aerial position, and, with a spring, slide it down the back of the supporting leg, bringing the other foot quickly to third aerial position. Repeat as required. This movement may also be executed starting or finishing in third rear aerial position. Each back-step occupies one beat of music.

Shuffle

Starting with one foot in mid-fourth aerial position low, spring or hop and, during the elevation, extend the original supporting foot to mid-fourth aerial position low. Then, almost simultaneously on landing, brush the new working foot inwards on the half point in third or fifth position and immediately brush it outwards to mid-fourth aerial position low.

Note 1: The inward brush is finished without the working foot losing contact with the ground and with the instep slightly relaxed to bring the heel over the instep of the support-ing foot, a position referred to as *'over the buckle'*.

Note 2: Shuffles are executed without lateral or forward travel but, where specified, a slight backward travel is used.

Note 3: If the movement preceding a series of shuffles finishes with the working foot in an aerial position other than starting aerial position given above, the first shuffle of the series is started from there.

Note 4: When, under certain stated circumstances such as are given in the first note in the Seann Triubhas description, it is necessary to start the first of a series of shuffles with a hop instead of a spring, there is no change of supporting foot during that shuffle as both the inward and the outward brushes are executed with the starting foot.

Examples for Counting (Four Shuffles)

(a) To Strathspey tempo 1& 2& 3& 4&

(b) To Reel tempo   1 & 2 & 3 & 4 &

Spring point

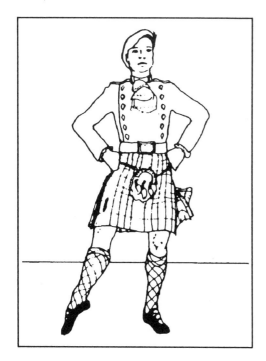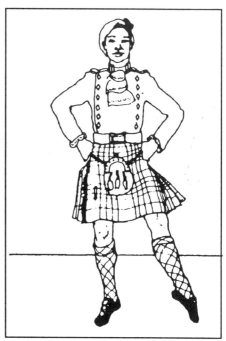

54/55

Spring, and point the working foot in an accepted open position, both feet touching the ground (54,55).

Pivot turn

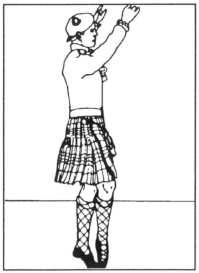

56

(a) Turning to the left: Take the right foot to the third crossed position on the half point pivot to the left on the balls of both feet without displacing them (56), finishing in third or fifth position with the left foot in front.

(b) Turning to the right: As above, but starting with the left foot and finishing with the right foot in front.

Note: The working foot may be extended to fourth intermediate aerial position before starting the pivot turn.

Note: Prior to placing-in third crossed position a small step backwards may be taken with rear foot. There is no extension to 4th intermediate aerial position in this method.

Hop-brush-beat-beat

Hop, extending the working foot to fourth intermediate aerial position if not already so placed, then quickly execute an inward brush to third aerial position low (count '1 and [and]'); place the working foot on the half point in third or fifth position then lightly beat the rear foot in third or fifth rear position (count 'a 2').

Note 1: Simultaneously on executing the beat with the rear foot on the count of '2', the working foot may be extended to fourth intermediate aerial position or second aerial position according to the starting position required for the movement which is to follow.

Note 2: The movement can also be executed to the count '5 and [and] a 6'.

Shake-shake-down

Hop, executing a shake action with the working foot in fourth intermediate aerial position; hop, carrying the working foot slightly backwards to execute another shake action with that foot in second aerial position then spring to displace the supporting foot which, if required is sharply extended to any open aerial position to start the next movement or taken to third aerial position very low prior to a quick step.

If desired, both shake actions may be executed in second aerial position in which case there is no backward movement of the working foot during the two shake actions.

Note: The starting position of the working foot depends upon whether or not it has been extended to finish the hop-brush-beat-beat movement by which it is invariably preceded.

Examples for Counting '3 & 4' or '7 & 8'

28

Propelled pivot turn

Danced during a Reel by two dancers, facing in opposite directions with the shoulder-lines parallel. The *inner arm* of each dancer is extended diagonally forward and linked with that of the partner, the *outer arm* being in second position, and the head turned slightly towards partner.

Note: 'The inner arms linked'—The inner forearms rest parallel and are in contact with each other, with the palm of the hand lightly supporting the underside of partner's arm just above the elbow. Since this is not a grip but an aid to balance, the thumb must not encircle partner's upper arm.

When danced turning to the right, the movement is begun by the partners moving forward with a slight spring on to the right foot whilst linking their right arms and adopting the position described above (count '1'); they now place the left foot on the half point in second position, to allow for a slight travel of the right foot (count '& 2'); the turn is now continued by repeating the actions described for the count of '& 2' as often as required (count '& 3 & 4', etc.) so that, while the right foot takes the main weight of the body, the left foot acts as a propelling force to produce the turn, during which the knees must be slightly relaxed. When danced turning to the left, the movement is begun by moving forward on to the left foot whilst linking left arms; the left foot then becomes the main supporting foot with the right foot providing the propelling force.

Progressive strathspey movement

Beginning with the right foot in third aerial position, step with that foot along the line of travel to fourth intermediate position (count '1'); close the ball of the left foot to fifth rear position, extending the right foot to fourth intermediate aerial position (count '2'); spring on the right foot along the line of travel bringing the left foot to third rear aerial position (count '3'); hop RF with slight forward travel, executing a round-the-leg movement with LF to third aerial position (count '4').

Note: On the first two counts the body is at an angle of 45° to the line of travel with the right shoulder leading; on the third count, the body faces the line of travel; on the fourth count, the body is at an angle of 45° to the line of travel with the left shoulder leading. This movement is executed with the opposite foot.

The head is always directed along the line of travel.

Progressive reel movement

Hop on the left foot taking the right foot to third aerial position, then step with the right foot along the line of travel to fourth intermediate position (count '&1'); close the ball of the left foot to third or fifth rear position then step with the right foot along the line of travel (count '& 2').

This movement is executed with the opposite foot.

Note: The body is used as for the progressive strathspey movement, beginning to change the shoulder lead on the step which precedes the hop.

C: Basic steps

A basic step is a combination of basic movements.

A detailed description of the steps which may be used in Championship Highland Dances is given in chapter two.

CHAPTER TWO: HIGHLAND DANCES

A Dance is a combination of a number of basic steps. In the following descriptions of the Dances the following abbreviations are used: RF = Right foot. LF = Left foot.

All dances should be preceded by an introduction of four bars of music except when the Reel of Tulloch is performed as a separate dance in which case it has an eight-bar introduction. Consequently there are sixteen counts in the introduction to each Highland Dance, the dancers standing during the first eight counts and bowing during the second eight.

With reference to foot work only, where fifth position is used in describing a step in any dance, third position may be substituted but, throughout that step, the same position–third or fifth–should be used.

In each of the following dances, the first and last steps given should always be performed as such, an exception being the Seann Triubhas, in which any of the quick steps may be used as a last step. The other steps may be performed in a different numerical order to that given in this book.

As a signal for the piper to change from slow to quick tempo the dancer <u>must</u> clap hands on the last beat of the slow step.

1: THE HIGHLAND FLING

A solo dance consisting normally of six or eight steps danced without travel except where specially mentioned in the alternative to the sixth (cross-over) step.

Music: ' Monymusk' or any other suitable Strathspey tune.

Tempo: $\downarrow$ = 124 (or 31 Bars to the minute).

The working foot is never placed in fourth position during the dance. The arms, when changing from one position to another, arrive at the new position on the first beat of the bar, except where specially mentioned in the sixth (cross-over) step.

Note: In the following description, the beginning of each step is given on the assumption that the steps are being performed in the numerical order given, but, should the order be varied, the movement with which each step begins (hop or spring) is determined by the finishing position of the preceding step.

INTRODUCTION

Bars 1 and 2: Stand as for bow.

Bars 3 and 4: Bow (count '1, 2, 3, 4, 5, 6'); may rise on balls of feet, taking arms to 1st position if not already so placed (count '7, 8').

FIRST STEP: SHEDDING

Bar 1: Commencing with disassemble on to LF, execute the shedding movement with RF (count '1, 2, 3, 4').

Bar 2: Beginning with spring RF (instead of disassemble), repeat bar 1 with the other foot (count '5, 6, 7, 8').

Bar 3: Beginning with spring LF (instead of disassemble), repeat bar 1 (count '1, 2, 3,4').

Bar 4: Beginning with spring RF, execute the shedding movement with LF but make a complete turn to the right while executing the three hops (count ' 5, 6, 7, 8').

ARMS: Second position in bars 1, 2, and 3; first or second position in bar 4.

Bars 5 to 8: Beginning with hop RF (instead of disassemble), repeat bars 1 to 4 with the opposite foot, turning to the left on bar 8.

SECOND STEP: FIRST BACK - STEPPING

Bar 1: Hop LF, pointing RF in second position (count '1'); hop LF, taking RF to third rear aerial position (count '2'); hop LF, pointing RF in second position (count '3'); hop LF, taking RF to third aerial position (count '4').

Bar 2: Execute back-stepping, springing RF, LF, RF, LF (count '5, 6, 7, 8').

ARMS: Second position in bar 1; third position in bar 2.

Bars 3 *and* 4: Beginning with spring (instead of hop), repeat bars 1 and 2 with the opposite foot.

Bars 5 *to* 8: Beginning with spring (instead of hop), repeat bars 1 to 4.

THIRD STEP: TOE-AND-HEEL

Bar 1: Commencing with spring LF, execute the shedding movement with RF (count '1, 2, 3, 4').

Bar 2: Spring, then hop on RF, executing toe-and-heel movement with LF in fifth position (count '5, 6'); spring, then hop on LF, executing toe-and-heel movement with RF in fifth position (count '7, 8').

Bar 3: Repeat bar 2 (count '1, 2, 3, 4').

Bar 4: Turn to the right as in bar 4 of the first step (count '5, 6, 7, 8').

ARMS: Second position in bar 1; first position in bars 2 and 3; first or second position in bar 4.

Bars 5 *to* 8: Beginning with hop (instead of spring) repeat bars 1 to 4 with the opposite foot, turning to the left on bar 8.

FOURTH STEP: ROCKING

Bar 1: Hop LF, pointing RF in second position (count '1'); hop LF, taking RF to third rear aerial position (count '2'); hop LF, pointing RF in fifth position then hop LF, extending RF with shake to fourth intermediate aerial position (count '3 and [and] a 4' or '3 [and] and a 4').

Bar 2: Execute four rocks, beginning with spring RF (count '5, 6, 7, 8').

ARMS: Second position in bar 1; third position in bar 2.

Bars 3 *and* 4: Beginning with spring (instead of hop), repeat bars 1 and 2 with the opposite foot.

Bars 5 *to* 8: Beginning with spring (instead of hop), repeat bars 1 to 4.

FIFTH STEP: SECOND BACK-STEPPING

Bar 1: Spring LF, pointing RF in second position (count '1'); hop LF, taking RF to third rear aerial position (count '2'); execute a quick round-the-leg movement with RF to third aerial position, then hop LF, extending RF to fourth intermediate aerial position (count '&3'); hop LF, returning RF to third aerial position (count '4').

Note: The round-the-leg movement with the RF may be executed quickly following the count of '2' in which case the counting for the bar becomes '1, 2& 3, 4'.

Bar 2: Execute back-stepping, springing RF, LF, RF, LF (count '5, 6, 7, 8').

ARMS: Second position in bar 1; third position in bar 2.

Bars 3 *and* 4: Repeat bars 1 and 2 with opposite foot.

Bars 5 *to* 8: Repeat bars 1 to 4.

ALTERNATIVE METHOD

Bar 1: Spring LF, extending RF to fourth intermediate aerial position (count '1'); hop LF, executing a high cut in front with RF (count '2&'); hop LF, extending RF to fourth intermediate aerial position (count '3'); hop LF, returning to third aerial position (count '4').

Bar 2: Execute back-stepping, springing RF, LF, RF, LF (count '5, 6, 7, 8').

ARMS: Second position in bar 1; third position in bar 2.

Bars 3 *and* 4: Repeat bars 1 and 2 with the opposite foot.

Bars 5 *to* 8: Repeat bars 1 to 4.

SIXTH STEP: CROSS-OVER

Bar 1: Execute the shedding movement with RF (count '1, 2, 3, 4').

Bar 2: Hop LF, pointing RF in second position (count '5'); hop LF, taking RF to third rear aerial position (count '6'); softly passing RF through third aerial position and down in front of the supporting leg, spring on to that foot to displace the LF which is raised to third rear aerial position (count '7'); hop RF, pointing LF in fifth position (count '8').

ARMS: Second position, changing to second position on the other side on the count of '7'.

Bars 3 *and* 4: Repeat bars 1 and 2 with the opposite foot.

Bars 5 *to* 8: Repeat bars 1 to 4.

Note: In the following alternative method given for executing bar 2 in the above step, the same arm movements are used as those given above.

ALTERNATIVE METHOD

As for bar 2 above but simultaneously on landing from the spring with RF on the count of '7', extend the LF to second aerial position low.

Note: A slight lateral travel may be introduced by springing to third crossed position instead of displacing the other foot on the seventh count.

SEVENTH STEP: SHAKE AND TURN

Bar 1: Execute bar 1 of the fourth step.

Bar 2: Turn to right as in bar 4 of the first step.

ARMS: Second position in bar 1; first or second position in bar 2.

Bars 3 *and* 4: Repeat bars 1 and 2 with the opposite foot.

Bars 5 *to* 8: Repeat bars 1 to 4.

ALTERNATIVE SEVENTH STEP (DOUBLE SHAKE AND ROCK)

Bar 1: Beginning with hop LF (instead of disassemble), execute shedding with RF, as in bar 1 of the first step (count '1, 2, 3, 4').

Bar 2: Hop LF, pointing RF in fifth position then hop LF, extending RF with shake to fourth intermediate aerial position (count '5 and [and] a 6' or '5 [and] and a 6'); repeat (count '7 and [and] a 8' or '7 [and] and a 8').

Bar 3: Execute four rocks as in bar 2 of the fourth step (count '1, 2, 3, 4').

Bar 4: Turn to the right as in bar 4 of the first step (count '5, 6, 7, 8').

ARMS: Second position in bars 1 and 2; third position in bar 3; first or second position in bar 4.

Bars 5 *to* 8: Repeat bars 1 to 4 with the opposite foot, turning to the left in bar 8.

EIGHTH STEP: LAST SHEDDING

Bar 1: Beginning with hop LF (instead of disassemble) execute the shedding movement with RF (count '1, 2, 3, 4').

Bars 2 *and* 3: Repeat bar 1 twice (count '5, 6, 7, 8, 1, 2, 3, 4').

Bar 4: Turn to the right as in bar 4 of the first step (count '5, 6, 7, 8').

ARMS: Second position in bars 1, 2 and 3: first or second position in bar 4.

Bar 5: Execute bar 5 of the first step, shedding with LF (count '1, 2, 3, 4').

Bar 6: Repeat bar 5 (count '5, 6, 7, 8').

Bar 7: Turn to the left as in bar 8 of the first step (count '1, 2, 3, 4').

Bar 8: Repeat bar 7 (count '5, 6, 7, 8').

ARMS: Second position in bars 5 and 6; first or second position in bars 7 and 8.

Bars 1 to 6: As for above (shedding three times with RF, then turn; shedding twice with LF).

Bar 7: Repeat bar 6 (shedding with LF).

Bar 8: Turn to the left as in bar 8 of the first step.

FINISH

Step to the right with RF and close LF to first position (flat) and bow.

2: THE SWORD DANCE (GILLIE CHALIUM)

A solo dance consisting of not more than five or six steps, the last of which is danced to a quick tempo but, when at least four steps are used, the second last step may also be danced to a quick tempo.

MUSIC: 'Gilllie Chalium'

Tempo 1 (Slow): ♩ = 116 (or 29 bars to the minute)

Tempo 2 (Quick): ♩ = 144 (or 36 bars to the minute)

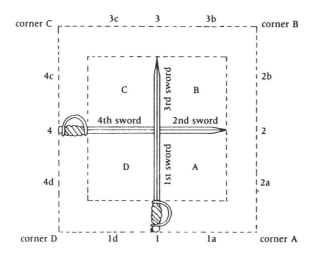

The dance is performed round and over two Highland broadswords placed crosswise on the ground at right angles to each other. The top sword is in a direct line from front to back with the hilt (called the top hilt) towards the dancer and with the centre of its blade directly above the centre of the blade of the other sword, the hilt of which is to the dancer's left. The hilts are placed as shown in the diagram but, when broadswords with a certain type of hilt are used, it may be found impracticable to place the hilt of the 'cross' sword as shown so that, in such cases only, that hilt may be placed facing the opposite direction.

Although only two swords are used it has been found expedient to refer to the half blade nearest the dancer's starting place (near the top hilt) as the First Sword then, working in an anti-clockwise direction, referring to the other half blades as the Second, Third and Fourth Swords.

In the diagram, two squares (an inner and an outer) are shown by dotted lines. The inner square embraces the sword blades which divide the square into four smaller squares termed 'spaces', the space on the right-hand side of the First Sword being denoted by the letter *A* and the other spaces, working in an anti-clockwise direction, by the letters *B*, *C* and *D*.

In the diagram, the spot on the ground approximately one foot-length from the top hilt and directly in line with the First Sword is denoted by the number 1, the corresponding spots on the ground in relation to the two sword points and the other hilt being denoted by the appropriate numbers. An outer square is depicted passing through the four spots and the corners are denoted by the letter corresponding to the adjacent space. To the right of spot 1, on the outer square and directly in front of the centre of space *A,* is the auxiliary spot 1*a* and the auxiliary spot 1*d* is to the left of spot 1 directly in front of the centre of space *D*. Similarly, the corresponding auxiliary spots in relation to the other main spots are denoted by the appropriate numbers and auxiliary letters.

Note 1: While dancing over or across the swords the head may be slightly inclined to allow the dancer to see the swords.

Note 2: When 'inside' the swords, the dancer should be placed in the centre of the space in which he is dancing or should be aiming to land in the centre of the space into which he is moving.

Note 3: When executing a Pas de Basque 'inside' the swords, there is no extension at the end.

Note 4: Where open Pas de Basque and spring point are mentioned in the description of the following steps, the supporting foot is given first.

Note 5: The amount of turn at the end of each step is determined by the starting position of the step which is to follow.

Tempo 1

INTRODUCTION

Bars 1 *and* 2: Stand at 1 as for the bow.

Bars 3 *and* 4: Bow (count '1, 2, 3, 4') ; step to 1*d* with LF and point RF in third position, (count '5, 6, 7'); pause (count '8').

Note: The dancer may rise on the ball of LF on the count of '8'.

OR

Bars 3 *and* 4: Bow (count 1, 2, 3, 4, 5, 6). Rise simultaneously on the balls of two feet on counts 7, 8 or place RF in third or fifth position on the half point keeping LF flat (count 7, 8).

FIRST STEP: ADDRESSING THE SWORDS

Bar 1: Pas de Basque with RF to 1a (count '1& 2'); Pas de Basque with LF to 1d (count '3& 4')

Bar 2: Make three-quarters of a turn to the right with two Pas de Basque, the first with RF to corner A, the second with LF at corner A without travel (count '5& 6, 7&, 8').

Bar 3: Pas de Basque with RF to slightly beyond 2 (count '1& 2'); travelling slightly to the left, assemble at 2 with RF in fifth position (count '3'); disassemble on to LF executing a high cut with RF (count '4&').

Bar 4: Execute four high cuts at 2, springing RF , LF , RF , LF (count '5& 6& 7& 8&').

ARMS: First position in bars 1, 2 and 3, changing to third position on the fourth count of bar 3; third position in bar 4.

Note: Where primary, Beginner sections are concerned, the dancer may omit the assemble and disassemble with high cut described in bar 3 above and substitute a Pas de Basque with LF to 2 (count '3& 4") in which case the arms are retained in first position for that Pas de Basque then raised to third position for bar 4.

Bars 5 to 8: As for bars 1 to 4, starting at 2 and finishing at 3.
Bars 9 to 12: As above, starting at 3 and finishing at 4.
Bars 13 to 16: As above, starting at 4 and finishing at 1.

SECOND STEP: OPEN PAS DE BASQUE
Bar 1: Pas de Basque into *A* with RF (count '1& 2'); Pas de Basque into *D* with LF (count '3& 4').
Bar 2: Open Pas de Basque into *A* with RF, LF fourth-opposite-fifth position in *B* (count '5& 6'); open Pas de Basque into *D* with LF, RF fourth-opposite-fifth position in *C* (count '7& 8').
Bar 3: Repeat bar 2 (count '1& 2, 3& 4').
Bar 4: Execute four spring points turning over the second sword, RF in *A*, LF fourth position in *B* (count '5'); with half turn to right, LF in *B*, RF fourth position in *A* (count '6'); with one-eighth turn to right, RF in *B*, LF fourth intermediate position in *A* (count '7'); with one-eighth turn to right, LF in *A*, RF second position in *B* (count '8').
ARMS: First position in bar 1; third position in bars 2 and 3; first position in bar 4.
Bars 5 to 8: As for bars 1 to 4, finishing with the spring points turning over the third sword.
Bars 9 to 12: As for bars 1 to 4, finishing with the spring points turning over the fourth sword.
Bars 13 to 16: As for bars 1 to 4, finishing with the spring points turning over the first sword.
Note: If the third (toe-and-heel) step or the seventh (quick) or eighth (quick) step with the alternative method for the first bar is to follow, then, on the last spring point in bar 16, make three-eighths turn to the right finishing LF in *D*, RF fourth position in *A*.

THIRD STEP: TOE-AND-HEEL
Begun with the dancer facing *A* with LF (supporting foot) in *D*, RF pointed in fifth position or pointed in fourth position in *A*.
Bar 1: Spring, then three hops RF in *D*, while executing the toe-and-heel movement twice with the working foot (LF) fourth-opposite-fifth position in *A* (count '1, 2, 3, 4').
Bar 2: Repeat bar 1 reversing the positions of the feet (count '5, 6, 7, 8').
Bar 3: With quarter turn to left on the first count, spring into *A* with RF, then hop RF, in *A*, executing one toe-and-heel movement with LF in fifth position (count '1, 2'); spring, then hop LF in *A*, executing one toe-and-heel movement with RF in fifth position (count '3, 4').
Bar 4: Execute four spring points over the second sword, each with the supporting foot in *A* and the working foot fourth position in *B* (count '5, 6, 7, 8').
ARMS: Second position in bar 1; second position in bar 2; first position in bar 3; third position in bar 4.
Bars 5 to 8: As for bars 1 to 4, finishing over the third Sword.
Bars 9 to 12: As for bars 1 to 4, finishing over the fourth sword.
Bars 13 and 14: As for bars 1 and 2 (over the fourth sword).
Bar 15: Travelling straight forward in a line parallel to the first sword and commencing to turn to the right, Pas de Basque with RF to 1*d* (count '1& 2'); assemble at 1*d* completing a half turn to finish facing the fourth sword with RF in fifth position (count '3'); disassemble on to LF with high cut RF (count '4&').
Bar 16: Travelling to the right on the first spring, execute four high cuts at 1, springing RF, LF, RF, LF (count '5& 6& 7& 8&').

FIRST ALTERNATIVE METHOD (For bars 15 *and* 16)

Bar 15: As for bar 3, but in *D*.

Bar 16: Execute four spring points over the first sword, turning as described for bar 16 of the second step.

Note: The note to the second step applies with reference to the seventh and eighth (quick) steps.

SECOND ALTERNATIVE METHOD (For bars 15 *and* 16)

To be used only as a lead into the seventh or eight (quick) step started by using the alternative method of executing bar 1.

Bars 15 *and* 16: As for bars 3 and 4, finishing over the first sword.

FOURTH STEP: POINTING

Bar 1: Pas de Basque into *A* with RF (count '1& 2'); Pas de Basque into *D* with LF (count '3& 4').

Bar 2: Spring point with RF in *A*, LF second position in *D* (count '5'); hop RF, pointing LF in fifth position (count '6'); hop RF, pointing LF fourth position in *B* (count '7'); hop RF, bringing LF back to point it in fifth position (count '8').

Bar 3: Spring point with LF in *D*, RF second position in *A* (count '1'); hop LF, pointing RF in fifth position (count '2'); hop LF, pointing RF fourth position in *C* (count '3'); hop LF, bringing RF back to point it in fifth position (count '4').

Bar 4: Spring point with RF in *A*, LF second position in *D* (count '5'); with quarter turn to left, hop RF pointing LF in fifth position (count '6'); spring point with LF in *A*, RF second position in *B* (count '7'); hop LF, bringing RF back to point it in fifth position (count '8').

ARMS: First position in bar 1; to second position on count '5' in bar 2, changing them to second position on the other side on count '1' in bar 3; first position in bar 4 or, alternatively, second position, changing to second position on the other side on count '7'.

Bars 5 *to* 8: As for bars 1 to finishing in *B*.

Bars 9 *to* 12: As for bars 1 to 4 finishing in *C*.

Bars 13 *to* 16: As for bars 1 to 4 finishing in *D*.

Note: If this step is to be followed by the third step or by the seventh or eighth step with the alternative method for the first bar, then bar 16 should be executed as follows: spring point into *D* with RF, LF second position in *C* (count '5'); hop RF, pointing LF in fifth position (count '6'); spring point with LF in *D*, RF fourth position in *A* (count '7'); hop LF, bringing RF back to point it in fifth position (count '8').

FIFTH STEP: DIAGONAL POINTS

Bar 1: Pas de Basque in *A* with RF, then into *D* with LF as in bar 1 of the fourth step (count '1& 2, 3& 4').

Bar 2: Open Pas de Basque into *A* with RF, LF fourth-opposite-fifth position in *B* (count '5& 6'); spring point with LF in *D*, RF fourth intermediate position in *B* (count '7'); spring point with RF in *A*, LF fourth intermediate position in *C* (count '8').

Bar 3: Open Pas de Basque into *D* with LF, RF fourth-opposite-fifth position in *C* (count '1& 2'); spring point with RF in *A*, LF fourth intermediate position in *C* (count '3'); spring point with LF in *D*, RF fourth intermediate position in *B* (count '4').

Bar 4: Beginning with spring into *A* with RF, execute four spring points turning over the second sword as in bar 4 of the second step (count '5, 6, 7, 8').

ARMS: First position in bar 1; third position in bars 2 and 3; first position in bar 4.

Bars 5 to 8: As for bars 1 to 4 finishing with the spring points turning over the third sword.

Bars 9 to 12: As for bars 1 to 4 finishing with the spring points turning over the fourth sword.

Bars 13 to 16: As for bars 1 to 4 finishing with the spring points turning over the first sword.

Note: The note to the second step applies also to this step.

SIXTH STEP: REVERSE POINTS

Bar 1: Pas de Basque into *A* with RF, then into *D* with LF, as in bar 1 of the fourth step (count '1& 2, 3& 4').

Bar 2: Spring point with RF in *A*, LF fourth intermediate position in *C* (count '5'); with quarter turn to the right, spring point with LF in *C*, RF fourth intermediate position in *A* (count '6'); with one-eighth turn to the right, spring point with RF in *C*, LF fourth intermediate position in *B* (count '7'); with one-eighth turn to the right, spring point with LF in *B*, RF second position in *C* (count '8').

Bar 3: Open Pas de Basque with RF in *C*, LF in *D* in fourth opposite fifth position (count '1& 2'); making a half turn to the right, open Pas de Basque with LF in fourth-opposite-fifth position in *D*, RF in *C* (count '3& 4').

Bar 4: Starting with spring into *A* on RF, execute four spring points turning over the second sword as in bar 4 of the second step (count '5, 6, 7, 8').

ARMS: First position in bar 1; third position in bars 2 and 3; first position in bar 4.

Bars 5 to 8: As for bars 1 to 4 finishing with the spring points turning over the third sword.

Bars 9 to 12: As for bars 1 to 4 finishing with the spring points turning over the fourth sword.

Bars 13 to 16: As for bars 1 to 4 finishing with the spring points turning over the first sword.

Note: The note to the second step applies also to this step.

Music changes to Tempo 2

SEVENTH STEP: OPEN PAS DE BASQUE QUICK-STEP

Bar 1: Pas de Basque into *A* with RF (count '1& 2'); Pas de Basque into *D* with LF (count '3& 4').

Bar 2: Open Pas de Basque into *A* with RF, LF fourth-opposite-fifth position in *B* (count '5& 6'); Open Pas de Basque with LF in *A*, RF fourth-opposite-fifth position in *B* (count '7& 8').

Bar 3: With quarter turn to the left on the first count, open Pas de Basque into *B* with RF, LF fourth-opposite-fifth position in *C* (count '1& 2'); open Pas de Basque with LF in *B*, RF fourth-opposite-fifth position in *C* (count '3& 4').

Bar 4: Open Pas de Basque with RF in *B*, LF fourth intermediate position in *D* (count '5& 6'); Open Pas de Basque into *A* with LF, RF fourth intermediate position in *C* (count '7& 8').

Bar 5: Open Pas de Basque into *B* with RF, LF fourth-opposite-fifth position in *C* (count '1& 2'); Open Pas de Basque with LF in *B*, RF fourth-opposite-fifth position in *C* (count '3& 4').

Bar 6: With quarter turn to the left on the fifth count, open Pas de Basque into *C* with RF, LF fourth-opposite-fifth position in *D* (count '5& 6'); Open Pas de Basque with LF in *C*, RF fourth-opposite-fifth position in *D* (count '7& 8').

Bar 7: With quarter turn to the left on the first count, open Pas de Basque into *D* with RF,

LF Fourth-Opposite-Fifth Position in *A* (count '1& 2'); Open Pas de Basque with LF in *D*, RF fourth-opposite-fifth position in *A* (count '3& 4').

Bar 8: Open Pas de Basque with RF in *D*, LF fourth intermediate position in *B* (count '5& 6'); Open Pas de Basque into *C* with LF, RF fourth intermediate position in *A* (count '7& 8').

Bar 9: Open Pas de Basque with RF into *D*, LF fourth-opposite-fifth position in *A* (count '1& 2'); Open Pas de Basque with LF in *D*, RF fourth-opposite-fifth position in *A* (count '3& 4').

Bars 10 *to* 16: With a quarter turn to the left on the first count repeat bars 2 to 8.

ARMS: First position in bar 1, third position in bars 2 to 16.

ALTERNATIVE METHOD (For bar 1)

Open Pas de Basque with RF in *D*, LF fourth-opposite-fifth position in *A* (count '1& 2');
  Open Pas de Basque with LF in *D*, RF fourth-opposite-fifth position in *A* (count '3& 4').

ARMS: Third position.

It is now necessary to make a quarter turn to the left on beginning bar 2.

Note: If the dance is to finish with this step, bar 16 should be executed as follows:
  Execute four back-steps in *D*, springing RF, LF, RF, LF, travelling backwards in a
  curving line to 1*d*.
  ʌRMS: First position.

EIGHTH STEP: CROSSING AND POINTING QUICK-STEP

Note: The amount of turn given for any open Pas de Basque or spring point in this step is
  approximate.

Bar 1: Pas de Basque into *A* with RF (count '1& 2'); Pas de Basque into *D* with LF (count '3& 4').

Bar 2: With one-eighth turn to the left, open Pas de Basque into *A* with RF, LF fourth position in *C* (count '5& 6'); with one-eighth turn to the left, open Pas de Basque with LF in *A*, RF second position in *B* (count '7& 8').

Bar 3: With one-eighth turn to the left, open Pas de Basque into *B* with RF, LF fourth position in *D* (count '1& 2'); with one-eighth turn to the left, open Pas de Basque with LF in *B*, RF second position in *C* (count '3& 4').

Bar 4: With one-eighth turn to the left, spring point with RF in *C*, LF fourth position in *A* (count '5'); with three-eighths turn to the right, spring point with LF in *A*, RF fourth intermediate position in *C* (count '6'); with one-eighth turn to the right, spring point with RF in *A*, LF fourth intermediate position in *D* (count '7'); with one-eighth turn to the right, spring point with LF in *D*, RF second position in *A* (count '8').

ARMS: First position in bar 1; third position in bars 2 and 3; first position in bar 4.

Bars 5 *and* 6: Repeat bars 2 and 3 (count '1& 2, 3& 4, 5& 6, 7& 8').

Bar 7: With one-eighth turn to the left, open Pas de Basque with RF in *C*, LF fourth position in *A* (count '1& 2'); with one-eighth turn to the left, open Pas de Basque with LF in *C*, RF second position in *D* (count '3& 4').

Bar 8: With one-eighth turn to the left, spring point with RF in *D*, LF fourth position in *B* (count '5'); with three-eighths turn to the right, spring point with LF in *B*, RF fourth intermediate position in *D* (count '6'); with one-eighth turn to the right, spring point with RF in *B*, LF fourth intermediate position in *A* (count '7'); with one-eighth turn to the right, spring point with LF in *A*, RF second position in *B* (count '8').

ARMS: Third position in bars 5, 6 and 7; first position in bar 8.

Bars 9 *to* 12: As for bars 5 to 8, but begin over the second sword and finish over the third sword.

Bars 13 *to* 15: As for bars 9, 10 and 11, but begin over the third sword and finish over the second sword.

Bar 16: With one-eighth turn to the left, spring point with RF in *B*, LF fourth position in *D* (count '5'); with three-eighths turn to the right, spring point with LF in *D*, RF fourth intermediate position in *B* (count '6'); travelling backwards towards 1*d* spring RF, taking LF quickly to third aerial position (count '7'); execute one back-step springing LF and finishing at 1*d* facing the front (count '8').
ARMS: First position in bar 16.

ALTERNATIVE METHOD (For bar 1)
Open Pas de Basque with RF in *D*, LF fourth-opposite-fifth position in *A* (count '1& 2'); Open Pas de Basque with LF in *D*, RF in *A*, making a quarter-turn to the left to finish with RF in second position (count '3& 4').
ARMS: Third position.
Note: When both quick-steps are being danced, this method must be used to begin the last one.

FINISH
Step to 1 with RF and close LF to RF in first position (flat) and bow.
Note: In major competitions, if only one quick-step is required, the eighth step should be danced.

3: SEANN TRIUBHAS

A Solo Dance consisting normally of not more than eight or ten steps, the last two of which are danced to the quicker tempo.
MUSIC: 'Whistle ower the Lave o't'
Tempo 1 (Slow): ♩ = 104 (or 26 bars to the minute).
Tempo 2 (Quick): ♩ = 124 (or 31 bars to the minute).
Grace of movement of body and limbs, associated with precision in foot positions, is a characteristic of this dance. The full range of arm movements is employed with the steps in slower tempo, and the general impression given should be a graceful and flowing exposition of Highland Dancing.

In any Seann Triubhas step (or alternative method of performing same) where shuffles are executed only as a 'four-shuffle-break' in the fourth and eighth bars, the first shuffle in bar 4 should commence with spring or hop LF and the first shuffle in bar 8 with spring or hop RF.

LINKING OF STEPS
The first step (brushing) is invariably followed by the second step (side travel) and details as to how they are linked together are given in the dance description.

According to the step which is to follow, the finish of the last (eighth) bar of certain steps in the slower tempo is varied as detailed below from the method described in the dance description.
(a) When a step which finishes with a shuffle is to be followed:
   (i) by any step other than the sixth step (leap and high cut), the sixth alternative step (leap and shedding) or the eighth step (side heel and toe) then the extension of the working foot (RF) at the end of that shuffle, i.e. at the finish of the step, is to fourth intermediate aerial position.
   (ii) by a step started with a leap (e.g. the sixth step), the last inward brush with the RF is finished on the count of '8' with an assemble with the RF in third or fifth position.

(iii) by the eighth step (side heel and toe), the last shuffle stops when the RF is brushed inwards to third position on the count of '8'. Then, during the elevation for the hop with which the eighth step starts, the RF is extended towards second aerial position.

(iv) by a quickstep the last inward brush finishes in third position on count '8'.

(b) When a step which finishes with a pivot turn is to be followed:

(i) by a step starting with a hop then for that hop, a disassemble is substituted.

(ii) by the fifth step (travelling balance), then the RF is extended to fourth intermediate aerial position in preparation for the starting spring.

(c) When the fifth step (travelling balance) is to be followed:

(i) by a step starting with a leap, the finishing extension is omitted thus finishing with the LF in third or fifth rear position on the count of '8'.

(ii) by the eighth or any quick step, the finishing extension is omitted thus finishing with the LF in third or fifth rear position on the count of '8'.

Note: The seventh step (high cut in front and balance) and the ninth step (Double high cutting) can not be followed by a step starting with a leap but this does not apply to the alternative method for the seventh step.

Tempo 1

INTRODUCTION

Bars 1 *and* 2: Stand as for bow.

Bar 3: Bow (count '1, 2, 3, 4').

Bar 4: Step LF towards second position making one-eighth turn to the right, or pivot one-eighth turn to the right taking the weight of the body on LF (flat) (count '5'); step RF to fourth rear position (flat) to finish with LF pointed in fourth position (count '6'); stand thus, taking arms to fifth position then raise them up in front of the body to fourth position and carry them out to third position (count '7, 8').

Note: After the count of '8' there is a slight rise on the ball of the RF in preparation for the start of the first step.

FIRST STEP: BRUSHING

During the following three bars the dancer travels forward to complete a circle to the left (anti-clockwise), finishing at the starting point facing the front.

Bar 1: Spring LF, then three hops LF, executing an outward brush RF with each movement count ('1, 2, 3, 4').

ARMS: To fifth position on count '1' then, with a circular action, take them upwards to fourth position and downwards through third position on counts '2, 3, 4'.

Bar 2: Spring RF, executing an outward brush LF (count '5'); spring LF, executing an outward brush RF (count '6'); spring RF, executing an outward brush LF (count '7'); spring LF, executing an outward brush RF (count '8').

ARMS: In first position, or as for bar 1.

Bar 3: Spring RF, then three hops RF, executing an outward brush LF with each movement (count '1, 2, 3, 4').

ARMS: As for bar 1.

Bar 4: Execute four shuffles, springing LF, RF, LF, RF (count '5& 6& 7& 8&').

ARMS: First position.

Bars 5 *to* 8: Starting with hop instead of spring, repeat bars 1 to 4 with the opposite foot but in bars 5 to 7, make a circle to the right (clockwise).

Note 1: When, as is invariably the case, the second step (side travel) is to follow, the last shuffle in the 8th bar finishes with the inward brush RF on the count of '8'.

Note 2: When an outward brush is executed in conjunction with a hop, it is begun by taking the working foot to third aerial position very low during the elevation, and finished with that foot in fourth aerial position. The same also applies when an outward brush is executed in conjunction with a spring, but, in the latter case only, the working foot may be brushed straight forward through first position to fourth aerial position.

Note 3: The sequence of outward brushes executed with a hop or spring in bars 1 to 3 and bars 5 to 7 of this step may be varied.

ALTERNATIVE FIRST STEP

Bars 1 to 4: As for bars 1 to 4 of the first step but the finishing extension of the LF on the last shuffle in the fourth bar is towards second aerial position low to lead into a Pas de Basque.

Bar 5: Pas de Basque LF (count '1 & 2'); Pas de Basque RF (count '3 & 4').

ARMS: First position.

Bars 6 and 7: Repeat bar 5 twice more (count '5 & 6, 7 & 8, 1 & 2, 3 & 4').

Bar 8: Hop RF, then three springs LF, RF, LF executing four shuffles with arms in first position (count '5& 6& 7& 8&').

Note: Note 1 which follows bars 5 to 8 of the first step applies also to this step.

SECOND STEP: SIDE TRAVEL

Bar 1: Hop LF, extending RF with shake to second aerial position high (count 'and and a 1'); close ball of RF in fifth rear position (count '2'); step LF to second position and close ball of RF to fifth rear position or fifth position (count '& 3'); step LF to second position and close ball of RF to fifth rear position (count '& 4').

During counts '& 3 & 4' the dancer travels directly towards the left side.

ARMS: To fifth position on count '1' then with a circular action during counts '2 & 3 & 4' take them upwards in front of the body to fourth position thence through third position and downwards at the sides.

Bar 2: Repeat bar 1 with the opposite foot, travelling directly towards the right side (count 'and and a 5, 6 & 7 & 8').

Bar 3: Repeat bar 1 (count 'and and a 1, 2 & 3 & 4').

Bar 4: Execute four shuffles, springing LF, RF, LF, RF (count '5& 6& 7& 8').

Note: For the same reason as given in Note 1 under bars 5 to 8 of the first step, the last shuffle in the above bar finishes with the inward brush LF on the count of '8'.

Bars 5 to 8: Repeat bars 1 to 4 with the opposite foot.

THIRD STEP: DIAGONAL TRAVEL

Bar 1: Facing diagonally to the right, execute the hop-brush-beat-beat movement with RF (count '1 and [and] a 2'); travelling slightly forward in a diagonal line to the right, spring RF, executing an outward brush LF, then spring LF, executing an outward brush RF (count '3, 4').

ARMS: Second position for the hop-brush-beat-beat movement then first or third position for the brushes.

Note: The remarks in Note 2 to the first step, concerning an outward brush when executed in conjunction with a spring, apply also to this step.

42

Bar 2: Execute the hop-brush-brush-beat movement with RF , finished with or
without extension of the working foot on count '6' (count '5 and [and] a 6'); execute
a pivot turn to the left, finishing facing diagonally to the left (count '7, 8').
ARMS: Second position for the hop-brush-beat-beat movement, first or fourth
position during the pivot turn. If fourth position is used for the turn, the arm which
is being raised from first position is taken up at the side through third
position.
Bars 3 *and* 4: Repeat bars 1 and 2 with the opposite foot, travelling forward in a
    diagonal line to the left, and turning to the right with the pivot turn which is
    finished facing diagonally to the right.
Bars 5 *to* 8: Repeat bars 1 to 4, but finish facing the front.
Note: Because this step travels forward it must be followed by the fourth step,
    backward travel, in order to regain the starting position.

ALTERNATIVE THIRD STEP
Bar 1: Execute bar 1 of the third step (count '1 and [and] a 2, 3, 4').
Bar 2: Execute the hop-brush-beat-beat movement with RF finished with or without
    extension of the working foot on the count of '6' (count '5 and [and] a 6'); execute
    the shake-shake-down movement with RF making a gradual turn to left (count '7 &
    8') or a quarter to left (count 8').
ARMS: In second position, changing to second position on the other side on count
    '8'.
Bars 3 *and* 4. Repeat bars 1 and 2 with the opposite foot, and finish facing diagonally
    to the right.
Bars 5 *to* 8: Execute bars 5 to 8 of the third step.

FOURTH STEP: BACKWARD TRAVEL
Bar 1: Execute the hop-brush-beat-beat movement with RF finished without extension
    of the working foot on the count of '2' (count '1 and [and] a 2'); hop LF , taking
    RF to third rear aerial position (count '3'); hop LF , executing a round-the-leg
    movement with RF to third aerial position (count '4').
ARMS: Second position.
Bar 2: Execute the hop-brush-beat-beat movement (count '5 and [and] a 6'); execute
    the shake-shake-down movement with RF , finished by extending LF to
    fourth intermediate aerial position (count '7& 8').
ARMS: Second position, changing to second position on the other side on count '8'.
Bars 3 *and* 4: Repeat bars 1 and 2 with the opposite foot.
Bars 5 *to* 8: Repeat bars 1 to 4.
Note: Whilst executing the shake-shake-down movements in the above step, gradually
move backwards so that original position is regained at the end of the step. If not preceded
by the third step (diagonal travel) this step may be performed on
    the spot, i.e. without travel.

ALTERNATIVE FOURTH STEP
Bar 1: Execute the hop-brush-beat-beat movement, followed by the shake-
    shake-down movement as in bar 2 of the fourth step (count '1 and [and] a 2,
    3 & 4').
Bar 2: Repeat bar 1 with the opposite foot (count '5 and [and] a 6, 7& 8').
Bar 3: Repeat bar 1 (count '1 and [and] a 2, 3 & 4').
Bar 4: Execute four shuffles springing LF, RF, LF, RF (count '5& 6& 7& 8').
ARMS: Second position in bars 1, 2 and 3; first position in bar 4.

Bars 5 to 8: Repeat bars 1 to 4 with the opposite foot.

Note: Whilst executing the shake-shake-down movements in the above step, move gradually backwards so that original position is regained at the end of the step.

FIFTH STEP: TRAVELLING BALANCE

Bar 1: Execute the balance movement, springing RF , LF (count '1, 2'); spring RF to displace LF which is taken to third rear aerial position (count '3'); execute a round-the-leg movement with LF to third aerial position then hop RF , extending LF to fourth intermediate aerial position (count '& 4' or '&4').

ARMS: Third position.

Bar 2: Execute the travelling balance movement, beginning with LF (count '5& 6, 7& 8').

Bars 3 and 4: Repeat bars 1 and 2 with the opposite foot.

Bars 5 to 8: Repeat bars 1 to 4.

SIXTH STEP: LEAP AND HIGH CUT

Note: This step should follow a step which may be finished with the weight of the body equally distributed on the balls of both feet in third or fifth position.

Bar 1: Leap landing with RF in front (count '1'); disassemble with high cut RF (count '2&'); hop LF , executing a high cut in front RF (count '3 and [and] '); place RF on the half point in fifth position, then lightly beat ball of LF in fifth rear position, extending RF to mid-fourth aerial position low (count 'a 4').

Bar 2: Execute three shuffles, springing RF , LF , RF (count '5& 6& 7&'); beginning with LF execute the elevation as for shuffle but assemble with RF in front in fifth position (count '8').

ARMS: Circle arms outwards and upwards at the sides through third position to fourth position during the leap on count '1'; second position for the remainder of bar 1; first position in bar 2, or, alternatively,

First position during the leap on count '1' then, during counts '2, 3, 4', raise the arms outwards at the sides through third position to fourth position; during bar 2, take the arms outwards through third position then downwards to first position on count '8'.

Bars 3 and 4: Repeat bars 1 and 2 with the opposite foot.

Bars 5 to 8: Repeat bars 1 to 4 but in the last bar, the third shuffle is finished with the inward brush RF to third position on the count of '7' then the RF is placed on the half point towards fourth intermediate position and the LF closed to fifth rear position, simultaneously extending the RF if required, to the position for starting the next step (count '& 8').

ALTERNATIVE SIXTH STEP (LEAP AND SHEDDING)

Bar 1: Leap, landing with LF in front (count '1'); disassemble taking RF to third rear aerial position (count '2'); hop LF executing a round-the-leg movement with RF to third aerial position (count '3'); place RF on the half point towards fourth intermediate position, then close ball of LF to fifth rear position extending RF to mid-fourth aerial position low (count '& 4').

Bar 2: As bar 2 in the sixth step but travelling slightly backwards to regain starting position (count '5& 6& 7& 8').

Bars 3 and 4: Repeat bars 1 and 2 with the opposite foot.

Bars 5 to 8: As for sixth step.

ARMS: As described for sixth step.

SEVENTH STEP: HIGH CUT IN FRONT AND BALANCE

Bar 1: Hop LF, with high cut in front RF (count '1 and [and]'); place RF on the half point in fifth position, then lightly beat the ball of LF in fifth rear position, extending RF to fourth intermediate aerial position (count 'a 2'); execute the balance movement, springing RF, LF (count '3, 4').

ARMS: Second position on counts '1 and [and] a 2'; third position on counts '3, 4'.

Bar 2: Repeat counts '1 and [and] a 2' of bar 1 (count '5 and [and] a 6'); spring RF, taking LF to third rear aerial position (count '7'); hop RF executing a round-the-leg movement with LF to third aerial position (count '8').

ARMS: Second position on counts '5 and [and] a 6' changing to second position on the other side on count '7'.

Bars 3 *and* 4: Repeat bars 1 and 2 with the other foot.

Bars 5 *to* 8: Repeat bars 1 to 4.

ALTERNATIVE SEVENTH STEP

Bars 1 *to* 3: Execute bars 1 to 3 of the seventh step.

Bar 4: Execute four shuffles, springing LF, RF, LF, RF.

Bars 5 *to* 8: Repeat bars 1 to 4 with the opposite foot.

Note: Following each high cut in front, instead of lowering the working foot to fifth position, it may be placed on the half point towards fourth intermediate position and the rear foot closed to fifth rear position. To compensate for the resultant slight forward travel, and to regain line, the dancer travels backwards during the shuffles in bars 4 and 8.

EIGHTH STEP: SIDE HEEL-AND-TOE

Bar 1: Hop LF, extending RF to second aerial position during the elevation and taking it inwards to third aerial or third rear aerial position simultaneously on landing (count '1'); place heel of RF towards second position, then, momentarily taking the weight on that heel, place the ball of LF in fifth rear position, allowing the knee of the right leg to relax (count '& 2'); place RF on the half point towards second position, then place ball of LF in fifth rear position (count '&3'); place heel of RF towards second position then close ball of LF to fifth rear position as before (count '& 4').

ARMS: Second position

Note: During this bar the dancer travels directly towards the right side.

Bar 2: Execute hop-brush-beat-beat (count '5 and [and] a 6'). Execute shake-shake-down finishing in second aerial position (count '7 & 8').

Bars 3 *and* 4: Beginning with hop RF, repeat bars 1 and 2 with the opposite foot, travelling directly towards the left side back to starting point.

Bars 5 *to* 8: Beginning with hop LF, repeat bars 1 to 4 but a pivot turn to the left may be executed on counts '7, 8' in bar 6, in which case a pivot turn to the right is executed on counts '7, 8' in bar 8.

NINTH STEP: DOUBLE HIGH CUTTING

Bar 1: Execute the hop-brush-beat-beat movement with RF (count '1 and [and] a 2'); hop LF with high cut RF (count '3&'); hop LF with high cut in front RF (count '4&').

Note: The extension to second aerial position of the working foot incorporated in the high cut, may be executed either simultaneously on 'beating' the rear foot on the count of '2', or during the elevation for the hop which follows that count.

Bar 2: Execute the hop-brush-beat-beat movement with RF but finish with the weight evenly distributed on both feet with the RF in fifth position (count '5 and [and] a 6'); disassemble, extending both feet towards second aerial position during the elevation and land on RF with high cut LF (count '7&'); hop RF with high cut in front LF (count '8&').

Note: When executing the above high cuts in front, the extension is taken towards second aerial position.

ARMS: Second position, changing to the other side on the count of '7'.

Bars 3 *and* 4: Repeat bars 1 and 2 with the opposite foot.

Bars 5 *to* 8: Repeat bars 1 to 4.

Music changes to Tempo 2

TENTH STEP: SHEDDING WITH BACK-STEP

Bar 1: Hop LF, pointing RF in second position (count '1'); hop LF, taking RF to third rear aerial position (count '2'); hop LF, executing a round-the-leg movement with RF, to third aerial position (count '3'); execute one back-step with RF (count '4').

ARMS: Second position, changing to the other side on count '4'.

Bar 2: Repeat bar 1 with the opposite foot (count '5, 6, 7, 8').

Bar 3: Repeat bar 1 (count '1, 2, 3, 4').

Bar 4: Hop RF, pointing LF in second position (count '5'); turn to the right as in bar 4 of the first Highland Fling step (count '6, 7, 8').

Bars 5 *to* 8: Repeat bars 1 to 4 with the opposite foot and turning to the left on bar 8.

ELEVENTH STEP: TOE-AND-HEEL, AND ROCK

Bar 1: Spring LF, then hop LF (or two hops LF if required), executing the toe-and-heel movement in second position with RF (count '1, 2'); two hops LF, executing the toe-and-heel movement in fifth position with RF (count '3, 4').

ARMS: Second position.

Bar 2: Execute four rocks, springing RF, LF, RF, LF (count '5, 6, 7, 8').

ARMS: Third position.

Bars 3 *and* 4: Repeat bars 1 and 2 with the opposite foot.

Bars 5 *to* 8: Repeat bars 1 to 4.

TWELFTH STEP: POINTING AND BACK-STEPPING

Bar 1: Hop (or spring) LF, pointing RF in mid-fourth position (count '1'); hop LF, taking RF to third aerial position (count '2'); hop LF, pointing RF in mid-fourth position (count '3'); spring RF to displace LF which is taken sharply to third rear aerial position (count '4').

ARMS: Second position, changing to the other side on count 4.

Bar 2: Repeat bar 1 with the opposite foot (count '5, 6, 7, 8').

Bar 3: Repeat bar 1 (count '1, 2, 3, 4').

Bar 4: Execute four back-steps, springing LF, RF, LF, RF (count '5, 6, 7, 8').

ARMS: Third position.

Note: The back-stepping in bar 4 is begun from third rear aerial position.

Bars 5 *to* 8: Repeat Bars 1 to 4 with the opposite foot.

THIRTEENTH STEP: HEEL-AND-TOE AND SHEDDING

Bar 1: Hop (or spring) LF, pointing RF in second position (count '1'); hop LF, taking RF to third rear aerial position (count '2'); execute the heel-and-toe movement with RF (count '3, 4').

Bar 2: Beginning with hop, execute the shedding movement with RF (count '5, 6, 7, 8').

ARMS: Second position in bars 1 and 2.

Bars 3 *and* 4: Beginning with spring RF, repeat bars 1 and 2 with the opposite foot.

Bars 5 *to* 8: Beginning with spring LF, repeat bars 1 to 4.

FOURTEENTH STEP: HEEL-AND-TOE, SHEDDING, AND BACK-STEPPING

Bars 1 *and* 2: Execute bars 1 and 2 of the thirteenth step.

Bar 3: Execute four back-steps, springing RF, LF, RF, LF (count '1, 2, 3, 4').

Bar 4: Turn to the right as in bar 4 of the first Highland Fling step (count '5, 6, 7, 8').

ARMS: Second position in bars 1 and 2; third position in bar 3; first or second position in bar 4.

Bars 5 *to* 8: Repeat bars 1 to 4 with the opposite foot, turning to the left on bar 8.

Note: If the above is used as a last step, bars 7 and 8 may be executed as follows: spring LF, pointing RF in second position (count '1'); execute two turns to the left as in bars 7 and 8 of the eighth Highland Fling step (count '2, 3, 4, 5, 6, 7, 8').

FIFTEENTH STEP: BACK-STEPPING

Bar 1: Hop LF, pointing RF in second position (count '1'); hop LF, taking RF to third rear aerial position (count '2'); execute two back-steps, springing RF, LF, and finish with RF in third aerial position (count '3, 4').

ARMS: Second position on counts '1, 2'; third position on counts '3, 4'.

Bar 2: Starting with spring (instead of hop), repeat bar 1 with the opposite foot (count '5, 6, 7, 8').

Bar 3: Starting with spring (instead of hop), repeat bar 1 (count '1, 2, 3, 4').

Bar 4: Turn to the right as in the fourth bar of the first step of the Highland Fling (count '5, 6, 7, 8').

Bars 5 *to* 8: Repeat bars 1 to 4 with the opposite foot.

PREPARATION FOR THE FINISH

Method 1: On the last bar of the final step of the Dance assemble, without extension, with LF in front (count '5'); leap, landing with RF in front (Count '6, 7'); pause (count '8').

Method 2: On the fourth count of the seventh bar of the final step of the dance, assemble, without extension, with LF in front (count '4'); then execute bar 8 as follows:

Leap, landing with or without change of foot (count '5, 6'); leap, landing with RF in front (count '7, 8').

Method 3: Execute two turns to the left as in the eighth Highland Fling step (see note to fourteenth step).

Finish

Step to right with RF, then close LF to RF in first position (flat) and bow.

4: STRATHSPEY

A Dance performed by four Dancers.

MUSIC: Any Strathspey Tune.

Tempo: ♩ = 124 (or 31 Bars to the minute).

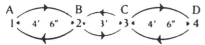

The set line is a imaginary straight line connecting points 1 and 4 thus passing through points 2 and 3.

As shown in the diagram, the four dancers A, B, C and D stand on the set line at points 1, 2, 3 and 4 respectively, A and B are facing each other C and D are also facing each other. As will be seen from the diagram, with reference to the line of travel, the term 'figure of eight' is a misnomer, but the name has been retained because it is traditional.

Note: The Strathspey is never danced on its own in competition, it must be followed by a Reel.

INTRODUCTION

Bars 1 and 2: All stand as for bow (8 counts).

Bars 3: All bow (count '1, 2, 3, 4').

Bar 4: All pivot one - eighth turn to the left on ball of LF , releasing the heel of RF (count '5'); point RF in fourth position, (count '6'); pause (count '7'); rise on ball of LF taking RF to third aerial position and raising the arms to third position (count '8'). OR, alternatively pause taking arms to first position if not already so placed (count '5, 6, 7'); rise on ball of LF swivelling to the left till the body is at 45° to the line of travel for the figure of eight taking RF to third aerial position and taking the arms to third position (count '8').

FIRST STEP: FIGURE OF EIGHT

Bars 1 to 7: Moving forward along the line of travel, as indicated by the arrows in the diagram, each dancer executes seven progressive Strathspey movements. Dancers A and D return to their starting positions at points 1 and 4 respectively; B and C, when approaching each other on the seventh bar, make approximately a three-eighths turn to the right, so that C finishes at point 2 facing A and B at point 3 facing D.

ARMS: Third position throughout.

Bar 8: Taking arms to first position, assemble with LF in front (count '5'); leap, landing with RF in front (count '7'); pause (count '8').

Note: During the figure of eight when A and D are passing each other in the centre, B and C are passing through the outer points, and vice versa.

FIRST ALTERNATIVE METHOD (For bars 7 and 8)

Bar 7: Execute the first three counts of the Strathspey movement with RF (step, step, spring), finished with LF in third rear aerial position (count '1, 2, 3'); gently extend LF to second aerial position with hop (count '4').

Bar 8: Taking arms to first position, assemble with LF in front (count '5'); leap landing with change of foot (count '6, 7'); pause (count '8').

SECOND ALTERNATIVE METHOD (For bars 7 and 8)

Bar 7: Execute the first three counts of the first alternative method above, then execute a round-the-leg movement with LF to third aerial position, followed by hop RF , extending LF to second aerial position (count '1, 2, 3 & 4' or '1, 2' 3 &4').

Bar 8: As for bar 8 in first alternative above (count '5, 6, 7, 8').

THIRD ALTERNATIVE METHOD (For bars 7 and 8)

Bar 7: Execute the first three counts of the first alternative method above, finished with LF in third rear aerial position (count '1, 2, 3'); taking arms to first position, assemble with LF in front (count '4').

Bar 8: Leap, landing without change of foot (count '5, 6'); leap, landing with change of foot (count '7, 8').

SETTING

Bars 9 to 16: All dance a Highland Fling step.

SECOND STEP: FIGURE OF EIGHT

Bars 1 to 8: As for bars 1 to 8 of the first step with B and C finishing in their original positions at points 2 and 3 respectively.

SETTING

Bars 9 to 16: All dance a Highland Fling step.

As it is essential to have the RF in third aerial position to start the Progressive Strathspey movement which is to follow the Highland Fling step used for setting, the last (8th) bar of Highland Fling steps which finish with the following move ments must be altered as described below:

Note 1: Bar 1 of all Highland Fling steps used for setting will begin with disassemble instead of hop or spring.

Note 2: On the last count of a setting step the dancers should make a one-eighth turn to the left preparatory to starting the figure of eight.

Note 3: If the Strathspey is to be followed by the complete Reel of Tulloch an even number of Strathspey steps should be danced, so that the dancers are in their original position to begin the reel.

LINKING OF STEPS

Back-stepping

On the last count of the step, hop LF retaining RF in third aerial position.

Rocking

On the last two counts of the step, spring LF, taking RF to third rear aerial position, then hop LF, executing a round-the-leg movement with RF to third aerial position or, alternatively, on the last count of the step, hop LF, taking RF to third aerial position.

The above also applies to the last setting step when the Strathspey is being followed by a Reel.

Cross-over

On the last count of the step, hop LF, taking RF to third aerial position, prior to Progressive Strathspey or Progressive Reel.

Highland Fling Turn

Following the completion of the last count of the turn, execute a round-the-leg movement with RF to third aerial position. This movement is not sharply executed and, when combined with the forward step that starts the Progressive Strathspey movement, give a perfect half-beat rhythm of '&1'.

This method does not apply when followed by a Progressive Reel movement, unless otherwise stated.

5: HIGHLAND REEL

This dance follows the Strathspey with the music changing to reel time without any break between the dances.

MUSIC: Any Scottish reel tune.

Tempo: $\downarrow$ = 108 (or 54 bars to the minute).

Note 1: During the Highland Reel the distance between the points may be reduced.

Note 2: On the last count of a setting step unless otherwise stated the dancers should make a one-eighth turn to the left preparatory to starting the figure of eight. An exception is at the end of the last basic reel step (high-cutting.)

FIRST STEP: FIGURE OF EIGHT

Bars 1 *to* 8: The dancers follow the same line of travel, and begin and finish at the same points as described in part 1 of the first step in the Strathspey, but eight progressive reel movements are danced to complete the figure of eight.

ARMS: Third position throughout

or, alternatively,

Execute seven progressive reel movements with arms in third position (7 bars); assemble with LF in front, taking arms to first position, then change (1 bar).

If this method is used, a basic reel step which is described as beginning with hop will instead begin with disassemble and, for a basic reel step described as beginning with assemble or the balance movement, preparation is made on the last count of the bar preceding that on which the basic reel step begins, by extending the RF towards second aerial position low or to fourth intermediate aerial position.

SETTING

Bars 9 *to* 16: All dance a basic reel step.

SECOND STEP: FIGURE OF EIGHT

Bars 1 *to* 8: As for the first step, but the dancers finish as for the second step of the Strathspey.

SETTING

Bars 9 to 16: All dance a basic reel step.

The first, or the first and second steps may be repeated using a different basic reel step each time.

When setting for the last time, all dancers execute the last basic reel step (high-cutting) to finish facing partners.

FINISH

All step to the right with RF, close LF to RF in first position (flat), then bow to partner. All step with LF into line facing the front, close RF to LF in first position (flat), then bow to audience.

6: BASIC REEL STEPS

FIRST STEP: PAS DE BASQUE

This step is performed by dancers A and D to start the Reel of Tulloch, the starting positions and the line of travel during bars 1 and 2 being given (a) on page 54 when the Reel of Tulloch has been preceded by the Strathspey and (b) on page 56 when the dance is being performed by itself.

Bars 1 and 2: Two Pas de Basque RF, LF, travelling forward towards set line to finish facing each other (count '1 & 2, 3 &4').

Note: The starting spring for each Pas de Basque is towards fourth intermediate position.

Bars 3 and 4: Two Pas de Basque RF, LF, making a complete turn to the right with A finishing at point 2 and D finishing at point 3 (count '5 & 6, 7& 8').

Bars 5 and 6: Pas de Basque RF, travelled slightly towards second position (count '1 &2'); assemble on the set line (A at point 2, D at point 3) with RF in fifth position (count '3'); disassemble on to LF with high cut RF (count '4 &').

Bars 7 and 8: Execute four high cuts, spring RF, LF, RF, LF (count '5 & 6 & 7 & 8 &').

ARMS: First position, changing to third position during the disassemble with high cut in bar 6.

SECOND STEP: SHAKE AND TRAVEL

Bar 1: Hop LF placing RF on the half point in fifth position (count '1'); hop LF extending RF with shake as for Highland Fling but to second aerial position (count 'and [and] a 2' or '[and] and a 2').

Bar 2: Hop LF, then step on to RF in fifth rear position (count '&3'); step LF to second position, then close ball of RF to fifth position (count '& 4') and then softly extend to second aerial position low.

ARMS: Second position, changing to second position on the other side on counts '& 4').

Bars 3 and 4: Repeat bars 1 and 2 with the opposite foot (count '5 and [and] a 6 &7 & 8' or '5 [and] and a 6 &7 &8').

Bars 5 and 6: Repeat bars 1 and 2 with extension to normal level before high cutting.

Bars 7 and 8: Execute two high cuts, spring LF, RF (count '5 & 6 &'); spring LF, taking RF as for high cut to third rear aerial position, then execute a round-the-leg movement with RF to third aerial position (count '7 &'); hop LF with high cut RF (count '8 &').

Note: On counts '7 &', the dancer may execute a high cut with RF instead of the round-the-leg movement described above.

ARMS: Third position.

ALTERANTIVE METHOD

Bars 1 to 4: Execute bars 1 to 4 as described above.

Bars 5 to 8: Execute eight high cuts with spring, beginning with spring RF (count '1 & 2 & 3 & 4 & 5 & 6 & 7 & 8 &').

ARMS: Third position.

THIRD STEP: BALANCE AND PAS DE BASQUE

Bar 1: Execute the balance movement, springing RF, LF (count '1, 2').

Bar 2: Pas de Basque RF (count '3 & 4').

ARMS: Third position in bar 1, first position in bar 2.

Bars 3 and 4: Repeat bars 1 and 2 with the opposite foot (count '5, 6, 7 & 8').

Bars 5 to 8: Repeat bars 1 to 4 making one-eighth turn on bar 8.

FIRST ALTERNATIVE METHOD

Bars 1 *to* 6: Execute bars 1 to 6, as described above.

Bars 7 *and* 8: Execute bars 7 and 8 of the second step.

SECOND ALTERNATIVE METHOD

Bars 1 *to* 4: Execute bars 1 to 4 as described above.

Bars 5 *to* 8: Execute bars 5 to 8 of the second step alternative method. (8 high cuts).

FOURTH STEP: BRUSHING

Bar 1: Hop LF , executing an outward brush with RF from third aerial position very low to fourth aerial position (count '1'); repeat hop LF , with outward brush RF (count '2').

Bar 2: Spring RF , executing an outward brush with LF from third aerial position very low to fourth aerial position (count '3'); hop RF , repeating the outward brush LF (count '4').

Bars 3 *and* 4: Execute four high cuts, springing LF , RF , LF , RF (count '5 & 6 & 7 & 8 &').

ARMS: Second position in bars 1 and 2; third position in bars 3 and 4.

Bars 5 *to* 8: Repeat bars 1 to 4 with the opposite foot.

FIFTH STEP: HIGH CUTS AND SPRING POINTS

Bar 1: Execute two high cuts, springing RF , LF (count '1 & 2 &').

Bar 2: Execute two spring points, springing RF , LF , with the working foot in fourth position each time (count '3, 4').

ARMS: Third position in bar 1; first position in bar 2.

Bars 3 *to* 6: Repeat bars 1 and 2 twice more (count '5 & 6 & 7, 8, 1 & 2 & 3, 4').

Bars 7 *and* 8: Execute four high cuts, springing RF , LF , RF , LF , with arms in third position (count '5 & 6 & 7 & 8 &') or, alternatively, repeat bars 1 and 2 (count '5 & 6 & 7, 8').

SIXTH STEP: BALANCE AND ROUND-THE-LEG

Bar 1: Execute the balance movement, springing RF , LF (count '1, 2').

Bar 2: Spring RF , taking LF to third rear aerial position, execute a round-the-leg movement with LF to third aerial position (count '3 &'); hop RF , extending LF to fourth intermediate aerial position (count '4').

Bars 3 *and* 4: Repeat bars 1 and 2 with the opposite foot (count '5, 6, 7 & 8').

Bar 5: Repeat bar 2 (count "1 & 2').

Bar 6: Repeat bar 5 with the opposite foot (count '3 & 4').

Bars 7 *and* 8: Execute four high cuts as in bars 7 and 8 of the fourth step (count '5 & 6 & 7 & 8 &').

ARMS: Third position throughout.

FIRST ALTERNATIVE METHOD

Bars 1 *to* 4: Execute bars 1 to 4 as described above.

Bars 5 *and* 6: Repeat bars 1 and 2.

Bars 7 *and* 8: Execute bars 7 and 8 of the second step.

SECOND ALTERNATIVE METHOD

Bars 1 *to* 4: Execute bars 1 to 4 as described above.

Bars 5 *to* 8: Execute eight high cuts with springs (count '1 & 2 & 3 & 4 & 5 & 6 & 7 & 8 &').

SEVENTH STEP: BACK-STEP AND TRAVEL

Bar 1: Take RF sharply to third aerial position and execute one back-step (count '1'); place LF on the half point towards second position (count '&'); place ball of RF in fifth rear position, extending LF to second aerial position (count '2'); take LF to third rear aerial position (count '&').

Bar 2: Spring LF with high cut RF (count '3 &'); spring RF, taking LF as for high cut to third rear aerial position (count '4'); execute a round-the-leg movement with LF to third aerial position (count '&').

Bars 3 *and* 4: Repeat bars 1 and 2 with the opposite foot (count '5 & 6 & 7 & 8 &').

Bars 5 *to* 8: Repeat bars 1 to 4 or finished with high cut RF.

ARMS: Third position throughout.

EIGHTH STEP: ASSEMBLE AND TRAVEL

Bar 1: Assemble with LF in front (count '1'); disassemble, taking RF to third rear aerial position (count '2').

ARMS: First position on count '1', second position on count '2'.

Bar 2: Hop LF, executing a round-the-leg movement with RF to third aerial position (count '3'); place RF on the half point towards second position (count '&'); close ball of LF to fifth rear position, extending RF to second aerial position (count '4').

ARMS: Second position.

Bars 3 *and* 4: Repeat bars 1 and 2 with the opposite foot (count '5, 6, 7 & 8').

Bars 5 *and* 6: Repeat bars 1 and 2 (count '1, 2, 3 & 4').

Bars 7 *and* 8: Execute four high cuts springing RF, LF, RF, LF, with arms in third position (count '5 & 6 & 7 & 8 &').

NINTH STEP: HIGH CUT IN FRONT AND BALANCE

Bar 1: Hop LF, with high cut in front RF (count '1 and [and]'); place RF on the half point in fifth position, then lightly beat the ball of LF in fifth rear position, at the same time extending RF to fourth intermediate aerial position (count 'a 2').

ARMS: Second position.

Bar 2: Execute the balance movement, springing RF, LF (count '3, 4').

ARMS: Third position.

Bar 3: Repeat bar 1 (count '5 and [and] a 6').

Bar 4: Spring RF, taking LF to third rear aerial position (count '7'); hop RF executing a round-the-leg movement with LF to third aerial position (count '8').

ARMS: Second position.

Bars 5 *to* 8: Repeat bars 1 to 4 with the opposite foot.

ALTERNATIVE METHOD

Bars 1 *to* 6: Execute bars 1 to 6 as described above.

Bars 7 *and* 8: Execute bars 7 and 8 of the second step.

TENTH STEP: SHUFFLE

Bar 1: Assemble with RF in front (count '1'); disassemble, taking LF to third rear aerial position (count '2').

ARMS: First position on count '1', second position on count '2'.

Bar 2: Hop RF, executing a round-the-leg movement with LF to third aerial position (count '3'); place LF on the half point towards fourth intermediate position, then close ball of RF to fifth rear position, at the same time extending LF to mid-fourth aerial position low (count '& 4').

ARMS: Second position.

Bars 3 *and* 4: Beginning with spring LF, and travelling slightly backwards to regain line, execute four shuffles with arms in first position (count '5 & 6 & 7 & 8 &').

Bars 5 *to* 8: Repeat bars 1 to 4 with the opposite foot.

LAST STEP: HIGH CUTTING

Bars 1 *to* 8: Execute sixteen high cuts, making a gradual complete turn to the right on the spot with arms in third position.

Note: It is not necessary to execute the high cuts with alternate feet. Double high cutting may be introduced by using a suitable combination of springs and hops. Furthermore, a round-the-leg movement may be substituted for one of the double high cuts. An example (starting with spring RF) is as follows:

Spring, spring, spring, hop; spring, spring, spring, hop; spring, hop, spring, hop; spring, spring, spring, spring.

7: REEL OF TULLOCH OR 'HULLACHAN'

MUSIC: 'Reel of Tulloch'

Tempo: ♩ = 108 (or 54 bars to the minute).

This dance usually follows the Strathspey as an alternative to the Highland Reel, in which case the dancers start in the same position as for the Strathspey, namely A and B facing each other at points 1 and 2 respectively; C and D facing each other at points 3 and 4 respectively.

Note: All high cuts performed during this dance are executed on the set line.

PART 1

Bars 1 *to* 8: Dancers A and D dance the first basic reel step (Pas de Basque).

Note: During bar 1 the forward travel is along the same line as for the figure of eight in the Strathspey or the Highland Reel.

During bars 1 and 2 of the above, dancers B and C, travelling forward and keeping to the left to pass dancers A and D, execute two Pas de Basque RF, LF with arms in first position (count '1 & 2, 3 & 4') or alternatively, two progressive reel movements RF, LF with arms in third position (count '&1 & 2, &3 & 4') to finish facing inwards at points 1 and 4 respectively, then stand in first position of the feet, arms and head for the remaining fourteen bars of part 1.

Bars 9 *to* 11: A and D dance the propelled pivot turn to the right, making approximately one and a half turns, finishing in a direct line with C and B (count '1 & 2 & 3 & 4 & 5 & 6').

Bar 12: Relinquishing the arm hold, execute two high cuts springing LF, RF, and making approximately a quarter turn to the right (count '7 & 8 &').

ARMS: Third position.

Bars 13 *to* 16: A and D dance the propelled pivot turn to the left, making approximately one and three-quarters turns (count '1 & 2 & 3 & 4 & 5 & 6 & 7'). Relinquishing the arm hold on the count of '7' continue the movement to finish with A at point 3 facing C, and D at point 2 facing B (count '& 8').

PART 2

(Starts B→   ←D A→   ←C)

Bars 1 *to* 8: All dance a basic reel step.

Bars 9 *to* 16: B with D and A with C dance the propelled pivot turn to the right, then to the left, as described in bars 9 to 16 of part 1, finishing with B and C facing each other at points 2 and 3 respectively, and with D and A facing inwards at points 1 and 4 respectively.

PART 3

(Starts $D\rightarrow$ $B\rightarrow$ $\leftarrow C$ $\leftarrow A$)

Bars 1 *to* 8: *B* and *C* dance a basic reel step.

Bars 9 *to* 16: *B* and *C* dance the propelled pivot turn to the right, then to the left, as described in part 1, *B* finishing at point 3 facing *A*, and *C* finishing at point 2 facing *D*. *A* and *D* stand for the above 16 bars in first position of the feet, arms and head.

PART 4

(Starts $D\rightarrow$ $\leftarrow C$ $B\rightarrow$ $\leftarrow A$)

Bars 1 *to* 8: All dance a basic reel step.

Bars 9 *to* 16: *A* with *B* and *C* with *D* dance the propelled pivot turn to the right, then to the left, as described in part 2, finishing with *D* and *A* facing each other at points 2 and 3 respectively, and *B* and *C* facing inwards at points 4 and 1 respectively.

PART 5

(Starts $C\rightarrow$ $D\rightarrow$ $\leftarrow A$ $\leftarrow B$)

Bars 1 *to* 16: *D* and *A* dance as described for *B* and *C* in part 3, finishing with *D* at point 3 facing *B* and with *A* at point 2 facing *C*.

B and *C* stand throughout in first position of the feet, arms and head.

PART 6

(Starts $C\rightarrow$ $\leftarrow A$ $D\rightarrow$ $\leftarrow B$)

Bars 1 *to* 16: All dance as for part 2 finishing with *C* and *B* facing each other at points 2 and 3 respectively and with *A* and *D* facing inwards at points 1 and 4 respectively.

PART 7

(Starts $A\rightarrow$ $C\rightarrow$ $\leftarrow B$ $\leftarrow D$)

Bars 1 *to* 16: As for part 3, but *B* and *C* finish in starting positions.

PART 8

(Starts $A\rightarrow$ $\leftarrow B$ $C\rightarrow$ $\leftarrow D$)

Bars 1 *to* 8: All execute the last basic reel step (high cutting) and finish as at the start, i.e. *A* facing *B*, *C* facing *D*.

Bars 9 *to* 16: *A* with *B* and *C* with *D* dance the propelled pivot turn to the right then to the left as before but finish *B*, *A*, *D*, *C*, facing the front at points, 1, 2, 3, 4, respectively.

FINISH

All stand in first position (flat) of the feet and bow.

Note 1: When begun from first position of the feet, a basic reel step which is described as beginning with hop will instead begin with disassemble and, for a basic reel step described as beginning with assemble or the balance movement, preparation is made on the last count of the bar preceding that in which the basic reel step begins, by extending the right foot towards second aerial position low or to the fourth intermediate aerial position.

Note 2: On the last count of a setting step unless otherwise stated the dancers should make a one-eighth turn to the left, preparatory to starting the propelled pivot turn. When the Reel of Tulloch is performed as a separate dance, the dancers begin as shown in the diagram.

$$B \rightarrow \qquad \leftarrow D$$
$$1 \qquad\qquad 2 \quad 3 \qquad 4$$
$$A \rightarrow \qquad \leftarrow C$$

REEL OF TULLOCH

A slightly forward and inward from point 1, facing *C*, who is slightly forward and inward from point 4; *B* slightly back and inward from point 1, facing *D*, who is slightly back and inward from point 4.

INTRODUCTION

Bars 1 to 4: All stand as above, ready for the bow (count '1 to 8').

Bars 5 and 6: Taking two small steps on the spot *A* and *D* make a quarter of a turn to the left while *B* and *C* make a quarter turn to the right to face partners in first position (flat) and bow (count '1, 2, 3, 4').

Bars 7 and 8: All return to starting position and acknowledge the dancer opposite with a modified bow (count '5, 6, 7, 8'). All follow the dance description given but during bars 1 and 2 of the first basic reel step which begins part 1, dancers *A* and *D* face and travel to points 2 and 3 respectively while, during Bar 1 dancers *B* and *C* step RF diagonally backwards on to the set line at points 1 and 4 respectively, close LF to RF in first position (flat) (count '1, 2') and stand thus for the remaining fifteen Bars of part one, with arms in first position.

CHAPTER THREE: RUDIMENTS OF MUSIC

Teachers and students should be conversant with the following musical terms and their definitions:

Staff
The five parallel lines and the four spaces between them upon, or in which the notes of the music are depicted.

Bar
The staff is divided by perpendicular lines called bar-lines, into short sections of equal value in the sense that each section takes the same period of time to play. The portion of music between any two consecutive bar-lines is termed a bar, which is itself divided into equal portions called beats.

Beat
One of the regular pulsations of the music, or one of the equal sub-divisions of a bar.

Time
The maintaining of a regular, or equal interval between beats.

Tempo
The speed at which the music is played, denoted either by the number of bars to the minute, or by a number giving the metronome time.

Accent
The emphasis placed on any particular beat. There are three accents in music, namely strong, medium and weak. The strong accent occurs only once in each bar, and always on the first beat of the bar.

Rhythm
The regular or periodical recurrence of accents.

Notation
The notes most generally used in music suitable for dancing are:

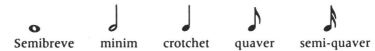

| Semibreve | minim | crotchet | quaver | semi-quaver |

The value of each of these notes is half the value of the preceding note, in the order given above, thus, taking the semi-breve as a standard, a minim is half, a crotchet a quarter, a quaver an eighth, and a semi-quaver a sixteenth of its value.

Time signature
The indication, at the beginning of the music, or any portion of music, which denotes the number of beats in each bar, and their value as a fraction of a semi-breve. When figures are used, the top figure gives the number of beats in the bar, and the bottom figure their fractional value (see notation).

Repeats
(a) The letters D.C., placed below the staff under a double bar-line, indicate to the musician to return, from that point, to the beginning of the music, the letters D.S., when

similarly placed, instruct the musician to return to the point in the music denoted by the sign S. .

(b) When a double bar-line is followed by two or four dots in the spaces of the staff, and the next double bar-line is preceded by two or four dots similarly placed, then the portion of music between these double bars is repeated.

Counting of Highland Dancing Steps or movement to music

It is essential that both the teacher and the student should understand the method of counting steps and movements to music, using the standard rhythms explained below, all of which refer to common time, since Strathspey and Reel tunes used for Highland Dancing are usually written with that time signature.

Note: In common time, which is denoted by the letter C on the staff, there are four crotchets in the bar, the accents being: strong, weak, medium, weak. Common time is the same as 4/4 time.

Single beat rhythm
Gives one sound in the space of time occupied by one beat. Thus there are four single beats in a bar of music (each represented by a crotchet) and counted:

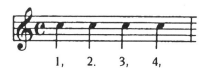

Half-beat rhythm
Gives two sounds of equal value in the space of time occupied by a single beat in the music. Thus there are eight half-beats in a bar (each represented by a quaver) and counted:

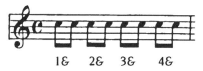

Imperfect half-beat rhythm
It has been found expedient to adopt the combination of (*a*) a semi-quaver, followed by a dotted quaver, with the beat falling on the semi-quaver, or (*b*) a dotted quaver followed by a semi-quaver, with the beat falling on the dotted quaver, as half-beats when counting steps or movements to music. Although neither of these combinations gives the sound of half-beats in a strict musical sense, since they are of unequal value, the semi-quaver being a quarter of a single beat, and the dotted quaver three-quarters of a single beat, the time-value of either of the combinations still equals the time-value of one complete single beat.

Method (a)
The beat falling on the semi-quaver is frequently found in music for Highland Dancing, the counting being denoted as follows:

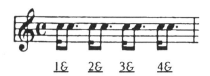

Method (b)
The beat falling on the dotted quaver is only occasionally found in music for Highland Dancing the counting being denoted as follows:

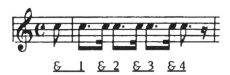

Triple beat rhythm
Gives three sounds of equal value in the space of time occupied by a single beat. Thus there are twelve triple beats in the bar (represented by twelve quavers grouped in threes, with that number depicted above each group) and counted:

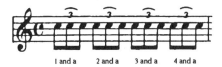

Note: In the dances described in this book, triple beat rhythm is not used in the counting of steps or movements to music, but it is widely used in other branches of dancing, good examples being the Irish Jig and Sailors' Hornpipe, which dances are frequently included at games or competitions.

Quadruple (or Quarter) beat rhythm
Gives four sounds of equal value in the space of time occupied by a single beat. Thus there are sixteen quadruple (or quarter) beats in the bar (each represented by a semi-quaver) and counted:

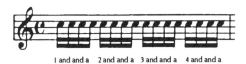

Note: When an' and' is shown in brackets, this signifies that there is no action by the dancer on that quarter beat, nor should it be sounded when counting.

NOTES
1 When denoting triple beat rhythm or quadruple beat rhythm, the writer deems it advisable to use the word 'and' fully written so that those rhythms may be quickly distinguished from half-beat rhythm and imperfect half-beat rhythm, in both of which the ampersand '&' is invariably used.
2 It is customary to group two consecutive bars of music together for the purpose of counting a step or movement, in which case the counting for those two bars–in single beats–would be 1, 2, 3, 4, 5, 6, 7, 8.
3 In any movement, when two actions are executed almost simultaneously (for example a 'spring point'), these actions are counted as if they were executed simultaneously, i.e. to one count.
4 When executing any movement of elevation, the dancer should land on the count, except on the few occasions where otherwise stated.

5 When the working foot has to be placed in or raised to any specified position while executing a movement of elevation, that foot arrives at the specified position simultaneously with the dancer landing on the supporting foot unless otherwise stated.

6 Although reel tunes are usually written in common time, they are played at a tempo so much faster than Strathspey tunes that it is found expedient to count steps or movements executed to Reel tunes as if the music were written in $\frac{2}{2}$ time, that is to say, counting two in the bar so that crotchets count as half-beats and minims as single beats. Consequently, for the same movements or steps, we get the same counting, no matter whether that movement or step is executed to Strathspey tempo or Reel tempo. For example, the counting for a Pas de Basque is 1 & 2, 3 & 4 whether that movement is danced to Strathspey tempo or to Reel tempo, yet that Pas de Basque occupies only half a bar when danced to Strathspey tempo and a complete bar when danced to Reel tempo.

SCOTTISH OFFICIAL BOARD OF HIGHLAND DANCING

Office Bearers
President   Dr. Alastair C. McLaren, T.D.
Vice-President   Miss Jessie Stewart
Chairman   Mr. Billy Forsyth

Examining Bodies
British Association of Teachers of Dancing
Scottish Dance Teachers' Alliance
United Kingdom Alliance of Professional Teachers of Dancing
Imperial Society of Teachers of Dancing

Represented Members
Highland Dancing Teachers' Association of England
Tayside Highland Dancing Association

Competition Organiser Members
Cowal Highland Gathering
Thornton Highland Gathering
Bute Highland Games
Duns Amateur & Athletic Cycling Club
Butlins Ltd
Stewarts & Lloyds Ltd: Recreation Club
Dumfries Highland Dancing Organisation
International Festival of Dancing and the Arts Society
Dundee Highland Dancing Association
Atholl Dancing Association
Harrow Festival of Scottish Dancing
Lancashire Festival of Highland Dancing
Caledonian Club of San Francisco
Glasgow Sports Promotion Council

Independent Members
Miss J. Stewart   Miss S. McDonald
Miss F. Paterson   Miss I. McKechnie
Miss E. McLaren   Miss W. Tolmie
Miss M. Rowan   Miss C. Orr
Mrs M. Todd   Miss B. Turkington

Honorary Members
Miss M. F. Lindsay   Miss S. Simpson
Mrs A. Duncan   Miss J. Ritchie
Miss`E. G. Strathern   Miss C. Tucker
Miss J. S. Keddie

Affiliated Members
Australian Board of Highland Dancing
Official Board of Highland Dancing (S A)
Highland Dance Teachers and Judges of Alberta
Pacific Northwest Adjudicators of Highland Dancing
Associated Judges & Teachers of Southern California
Professional Highland Dance Association (Ottawa, Cornwall and Montreal Area)
Professional Highland Dance Association (Toronto-Hamilton Area)
Highland Dancers' Alliance
Eastern United States Professional Highland Dance Association
Federation of United States Teachers and Adjudicators
Professional Highland Dance Adjudicators and Teachers of Western Ontario
Scotdance Canada
South Eastern United States Highland Dancing Association

Associate Members
Alberta Highland Dancing Association
Montreal Highland Dancing Association
Northern California Highland Dancing Association
British Columbia Highland Dancing Association
Manitoba Highland Dancers' Alliance
Ottawa Highland Dancing Association
Stormont, Dundas and Glengarry Highland Dancing Association
Highland Dancers' Association of Ontario
Eastern Canada Highland Dancers' Alliance
United Scottish Society of California
Perth Highland Games Association
Scotdance
Scottish American Society of Central Florida
Western Ontario Highland Dancers' Association

Acknowledgements
The late Mr. Harry Fairley for his generosity in giving the Board the use of his rooms and in providing films and still photographs, and particularly the Technical and Judges Committee, headed by Miss J. Stewart. To all members of the Board including our President, Dr. Alistair McLaren. To our Chairman Mr. Billy Forsyth, our Director of Administration Miss Marjory Rowan and to our late Vice President, Mr. William M. Cuthbertson, to whom we are all deeply grateful.

Copies of the Constitution and Rules can be obtained on payment from the Director of Administration, S.O.B.H.D., Heritage House, 32 Grange Loan, Edinburgh EH9 2NR.